My Brain Tumour
One Woman's Uplifting Story

Lynda K Carter
http://lynda-mybraintumour.blogspot.com/

Copyright © 2013 Lynda Carter
All rights reserved

Copyright © 2013 Lynda Carter

All rights are reserved including resale rights. No part of this publication may be reproduced in any form or by any means, including scanning, photocopying, or otherwise without prior written permission of the copyright holder.

Disclaimer
Please note that much of this publication is based on personal experience and anecdotal evidence. Although the author and publisher have made every reasonable attempt to achieve complete accuracy of the content in this Book, they assume no responsibility for errors or omissions. Also, you should use this information as you see fit, and at your own risk. Your particular situation may not be exactly the same as illustrated here; in fact, it's likely that they won't be the same, and you should adjust your use of the information and liaise with your physician accordingly.

Any trademarks, service marks, product names or named features are assumed to be the property of their respective owners, and are used only for reference. There is no implied endorsement if we use one of these terms.

Finally, use your head. Nothing in this Book is intended to replace common sense, legal, medical or other professional advice, and is meant to inform and entertain the reader. So please treat accordingly and good luck for the future.

ISBN: 1456312049
ISBN-13: 978-1456312046

ACKNOWLEDGMENTS

I wish to thank my sister, Sallyann Ewens, for her contribution to this book. Her version of events and emotions experienced added insight and humour. I also could not have done without her at my side.

DEDICATION

To my husband, Roy Carter. I know you didn't sign up for any of this but I can honestly say I cannot have wished to have had a better man by my side. Thank you and I love you very much. I know you don't like to be reminded but the memory is there and we came through it.

CONTENTS

INTRODUCTION

1. Let Me Set The Scene:
2. Wednesday 12th July
   MRI Testing.
3. Friday 14th July
   MRI Results
4. Friday 14th July
   Back To The Doctors
5. Friday 14th July
   Informing Family and Friends
6. Sat 15th July
   Visit To The Neurosurgeon
7. Sunday 16th July
   A Day To Ourselves
8. Monday 17th July
   Pre Operation Testing
9. Tuesday 18th July
   Blood Pressure Reading
10. Wed 19th July
    Operation Day
11. Thursday 20th July
    Intensive Care Unit

12. Friday 21st July

   Toy Town Ambulance

13. Saturday 22nd July

   Escape From ICU

14. Sunday 23rd July

   A Quiet Day Of Anticipation

15. Monday 24th July

   Sally Arrives

16. Tues 25th to Thurs 27th July

   Sally's Stay

17. Friday 28th July

   Sadness and Elation

18. Saturday 29th July

   Off Home

19. After Effects

OUR WEDDING DAY

My Sister Sally's Version Of Events

MY THANK YOU PAGE

Some Facts And Resources

INTRODUCTION

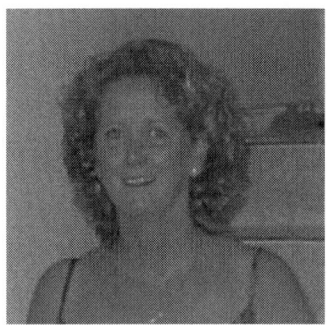

Hi,
My name is Lynda.

In some respects I'm sorry that you have found the need to purchase my book.

You are probably desperately searching for answers having recently been told that either you or someone very close to you has a meningioma. My thoughts and good wishes are with you all.

Your journey is just about to begin and the purpose of me writing this book is to share with you my journey in the hope that it will help you a little to understand the emotions, shock and sheer terror that such news brings and to offer some encouragement.

The one thing I have learnt though throughout my research is that nobody has the exact same experience and it is therefore my aim to include the resources to find good information and associations that have forums for you to ask questions of other meningioma survivors. Please remember what I said above though, that everybody has a different story and we all experienced different things. Your story will be different again and one of your best friends at this time will be your doctor. If you haven't already, find one that has time for you, one that you trust and respect and ask as many questions as you need to.

Being diagnosed with a brain tumour is a nightmare. It turns your world upside down and is both scary and worrying for both the victim and their family. I use the word 'victim', because that's how I felt at the time and I hope that by reading my story it will help you in coming to terms with your own situation.

My very happy world was hit by a thunderbolt on the 14th July 2006 when I was diagnosed with a brain tumour. I had a brain tumour; I had it surgically removed on 19th July 2006 and was back in my own home on 29th July, relieved that I had made it through safely, thankful for a second chance and wondering what all the initial fuss was about.

I don't mean to be flippant in any way. I know that I was probably luckier than most with regard to the position of my meningioma, I had a fabulous doctor with in-sight, I had a top rate neurosurgeon, I had my hero and the love of my life by my side, I had the love of family and friends and I also had the will and determination to overcome this hiccup in my life. I am a survivor.

QUOTE - Unknown Author
More powerful than the will to win is the courage to begin
.

1. Let Me Set The Scene:

My name is Lynda Burke. I am, at the time of writing, 48 years old. I have, so far, had a good life. I have travelled the world, lived in many different places; I have a supporting family that I love and some very loyal, caring friends who are great fun to be around.

Two years ago I immigrated to Cyprus, the island of Aphrodite and love. I settled into the Mediterranean lifestyle with my soul mate at my side and we decided to change the course of our lives completely. I left the drudgery of a 9-5 job and under the guidance of my partner, I learnt new skills, challenged myself and together Roy and I started a new internet business www.rent-a-villa-in-Paphos.com of which I am incredibly proud and which is now flourishing. I had everything and was immensely happy, in fact, happier than I had ever been in my life.

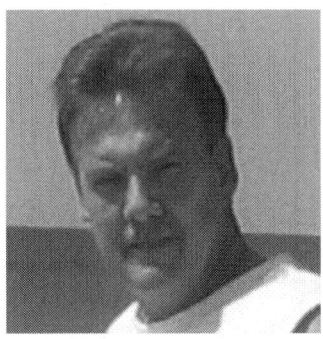

Roy Carter

My Brain Tumour

So, as you can see, life has been very kind to me. I have had very little sickness in my life and have never been in hospital for any reason other than to work as an admin clerk for 6 months. So, yes, you have it right, I have my tonsils and my appendix and I have never broken a bone in my body or had food poisoning or a baby. Remarkable isn't it that I escape a hospital visit for 48 years? But, boy, when I do it, I do it big! No messing around!

After waking up one morning in Mid June, I stretched, as you do at the start of a new day and at the end of this stretch my lower leg started to kick involuntarily at about one second intervals. Just to make sure you have the picture correct, I don't mean a kick that would score a goal, more of a gentle flick as if trying to get the sand out of your toes. I grabbed my leg and pulled it back to try and stop it, I got up out of bed and stood on it but that didn't work either. Now this in itself was a little scary and unpleasant – who likes to be out of control? Certainly not me! This little episode lasted all of 30 seconds, although it did feel like 10 minutes to me.

So, what was all that about? I thought I may have trapped a nerve in my back or hip. Why I thought that, I don't know. I have no medical training. It just seemed like a plausible explanation to me at the time.

Because of this self-diagnosis, I decided to put the incident on hold and see if it happened again, then if it became troublesome or painful I would see the Doctor.

Well, guess what? It took a few weeks, but yes, it did happen again. Just as before, I was in bed, but this time it woke me from sleep. Once again it lasted for approximately 30 seconds and worried me a little. I am ashamed to say that I let this happen twice more over a further period of two weeks and it wasn't until it happened at my desk that it suddenly dawned on me that I had to find the time, go to the doctors and get this trapped nerve sorted out. After all, this could happen in the supermarket or even worse while I'm driving!

On Tuesday, 11th July 2006 I went to see my doctor, Chris Theophanides. I told him my symptoms and then went on to tell him my diagnosis - he must have wondered why I had gone to see him! Well Dr Theophanides listened patiently to all my theories and then quite calmly told me he wanted me to have an MRI test of my head. (Magnetic Resonance Imaging - The MRI scan uses magnetic and radio waves, meaning that there is no exposure to X-Rays or any other damaging forms of radiation.)

Well this was strange. I have to admit to feeling slightly annoyed and frustrated. How did a twitch in my leg suddenly warrant an MRI test of my head? I asked him for his thought process and what he was possibly suggesting. He advised me that he thought the nerve twitch could be a neurological problem because there was also a tingling sensation around my knee. I have to say at this stage that I felt he was really over reacting and told him so but he felt it was better to start at the top when dealing with the nervous system and once he mentioned the 'epilepsy' word I felt slightly alarmed that the conversation was taking this turn. An appointment for an MRI test was made over the phone for the following day.

On the way back in the car Roy and I discussed what the doctor had said and I reiterated that I felt he was over reacting and that it was still going to be a trapped nerve in my back or leg. After all, I wasn't feeling unwell so what else could it be? However, Roy was concerned and therefore I happily agreed to go ahead because I was convinced it would show nothing and regardless of cost, I'd start at the top of the testing pile and take it from there.

QUOTE - Mark Twain
Get your facts first, and then you can distort them as you please.

2. Wednesday 12th July

MRI Testing.

We arrive at hospital for the MRI test. I am happy in the knowledge that this will all be a formality. The MRI equipment can be quite daunting to some people due to the confined space. All metal items must be removed. You are asked to lie on a bed and your head is positioned in a special holding device as it is imperative that you do not move while the equipment is in operation. The bed then slides into the cylindrical chamber of the machine and the room is emptied of everyone apart from you.

You will be handed a call button if you feel unwell or want the process stopped for any reason and be aware that even though you are alone, if you speak they will hear you. So do not feel that you cannot summon someone just because they are absent from the room. The machine then starts making a series of loud clicking noises and the procedure usually takes about 20-30 minutes.

The MRI technician explained the procedure and asked what my symptoms were. I was then positioned on the equipment and was feeling quite comfortable, best to shut your eyes and relax. About 15 minutes into my testing, all procedure stopped.

The door to the MRI room is opened and at this stage I am only able to see people from waste level downwards and therefore I am unable to see faces and my hearing is muffled by the head frame. A blue gowned person approaches me; he crouches to see me and asks my name. He explains that he is an anaesthetist but that he is not going to put me to sleep. He is simply going to put a cannula into my hand. I start to feel a little anxious and tell him that I will have no problem with him doing that as long as he explains why. The anaesthetist explains that the procedure is to enable a contrast dye to be injected into my system so that the image pictures are clearer.

My sense of all being well is rocked slightly as things seem to be happening quite quickly and with a sense of urgency on everyone else's part. At this stage I take a deep breath and have to be honest that I felt that something had been found and it wasn't good.

The rest of the test takes a further 10 minutes and during this I had to give myself a good talking to and try to think about it calmly. My first reaction was to try and convince myself that the contrast was probably quite a normal procedure in Cyprus but on reflection I feel this was more than likely denial of the truth on my part because nobody had mentioned the contrast before the test began.

I'm not sure at this stage if it's scary or not or whether in fact I actually want to know, but my heart rate definitely quickened and my chest tightened. I can't let my mind start wandering into dark, unknown recesses. I'd prefer to stick to the theory that the leg twitch is just trapped nerve damage.

MRI Testing

Once I'm off the machine and dressed again the Radiologist asks me to take a seat and asks what I'm feeling. It's very strange and once again I feel that everyone knows something that I don't. He asks if I am having any headaches and I say no, none at all. The feeling of frustration starts to take over again because I start feeling that no one is actually listening to me because the problem here is, as I have explained previously, in my leg and not my head and maybe they have someone else's notes!

That was basically the end of the conversation and I am left with a cold shiver running through my entire body. The alarm bells are ringing and I feel a wave of panic which I immediately stamp on as me being paranoid. Again, I tell myself that there is no point getting worked up until the results are through. What has the MRI radiologist seen? Why didn't I ask him? Surely if it had been something bad I would have been able to tell. Maybe he asked me the question because he couldn't see anything or nothing obvious was showing.

Anyway, I am told I can pick up the result the next morning, Thursday 13th and take the report back to my own doctor. That's it then. If they are letting me pick up the results all must be clear with no problems and I look forward to another set of tests which may find my trapped nerve.

Between you and me though, questions are flying round in my head all Wednesday night. Why did I have the contrast and why did he ask if I was having headaches? My solution to test the doctor's reaction was a simple one.

I decided I would phone Dr Theophanides, my doctor, on Thursday morning and tell him that as it was such a fabulous day I fancied going to the beach and would it be a problem if I picked my MRI results up on Friday and then came to see him. My rationale told me that if there was a problem he was going to say that he wanted to see me straight away. So I tested the theory the next day and Dr Theophanides said it was no problem at all, told me to enjoy my day at the beach and come in and see him at 10am on Friday. Surely, no problem then, you would think? Wouldn't you?

It's always strange to me in these circumstances how everybody is indirect with each other. Why didn't I ask the doctor on the phone outright if he had heard anything or if everything was ok? Why didn't the doctor ask how the test had gone or tell me that he had spoken to the Radiologist. Maybe he hadn't spoken to him at that time but it is the unspoken word that gets under the skin, starts crawling and sets the panic in motion. Very interesting! When something important is going on, silence would appear to be masking the truth.

Roy and I did exactly the same with each other at the beach that day. It was a curious day. I very much needed to be with Roy but I also wanted to be alone and didn't really know why. It was probably because I knew that if we sat on the beach and discussed our fears all day, I may actually have to confront them. We both knew all was not well. We are very close to each other and very much in tune with each other's feeling. The unspoken word between us was that we were both very worried and scared about what had happened yesterday. So, my little friend 'denial' came to the beach with us that day. I shut out the problems of tomorrow and tried to enjoy the day.

3. Friday 14th July

MRI Results

An appointment had been arranged with my Doctor, Chris Theophanides for 10am and as Roy had some work to do before hand, I decided that I would go down to the hospital on my own, pick up the results, bring them back home and then we could visit the doctor together.

Roy was obviously subconsciously feeling as anxious as me as he got out of bed early, finished his work in record time and told me he was coming with me.

We set off full of high spirits, joking around with each other as if we didn't have a care in the world. We didn't yesterday and we were not going to have today until someone convinced us otherwise. All thought of the contrast during testing on Wednesday was pushed well into the back of my mind. I look at Roy and wonder what he is thinking. If he thinks something sinister is going on he is hiding it well. I didn't make a big thing about the contrast and although the MRI technician had spoken to him to tell him of the process, I'm not too sure if he fully understood what happened there.

We are asked to take a seat in reception and after a short wait the Radiologist approaches us with the envelope carrying the MRI images. He smiles a welcome, then, he hesitates, looking a little unsure as he is just about to hand them over and says, "No. Can I ask you to come into my office?"

Whoa! Well this really spooked me out and made me take a really deep breath. What was happening here? Fear of the unknown was so horrendous in this short space of time between standing up and reaching his office; about 30 feet away. I felt hysterical and wanted to start laughing. My pulse was racing. I looked at Roy and he looked at me and I could see he was feeling exactly the same as me and that we were both thinking – Oh my God!

Once in the office the radiologist asked me to take a seat and explained to me that he had found the cause of my leg twitch and I said great! I sincerely meant great but had the feeling that a really big BUT was about to escape his lips. Everything seemed to freeze in time as if we were waiting for the answer to the 64 million pound question and the only thing that was going through my mind is this is really bad because he is holding images of my head in his hand.

I was seriously trying to keep it all together because it was important for me to listen. He has the facts in front of him and he wants to share them with me but, as he took the images out of the packet and switched the wall light on, I really didn't want him to put them up and show me.

Nevertheless, the gentleman has a job to do so he switches on the light, puts the images on the screen in front of me and says, "Lynda you have, and I want to completely stress here, a BENIGN TUMOUR which is sitting on top of your brain".

Oh, well that's ok then, breathe a sigh of relief.

I don't think so!

The word 'tumour' carries powerful shock waves. The word 'benign' took second place when it should have taken first. I was listening intently and I heard all he was saying but it was as if he was giving me bad news about someone else. I do not feel ill, I have no headaches or any pain but right at that moment I was scared for my life because I knew he was speaking to me, Lynda Burke, and I couldn't understand how this could be happening. I felt like I had just been handed a death sentence.

At this stage, I am sure I should have been feeling ecstatic that the tumour was benign. This is repeated again and again by the radiologist but I am still trying to process the first bit, which is the fact that I have a tumour on my brain. So, I have to swallow hard and stop myself from crying and becoming hysterical and tell myself to look at the pictures, look at the pictures Lynda and process the information.

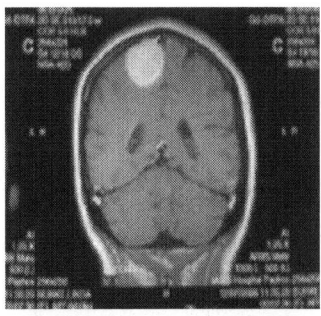

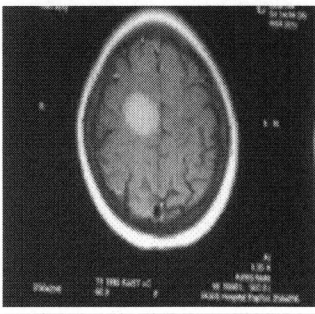

There, right in front of me, are very clear images showing a white egg on the top of my brain. It looks huge. How can something that big be growing in my head and not causing me any pain? It looks to me like the same size as a golf ball but is in fact approximately 3cm across.

The emotional rush had to stop while I concentrated hard to listen. I cannot think of a more challenging time. This very gently spoken Radiologist is telling me that I have what is called a meningioma, which is the most common type of tumour. It is sitting between the skull membrane and the brain. It is not penetrating the brain in any way but as it grows it is pushing against the brain, fighting it for space and causing a pressure which in turn is restricting the part of the brain function that controls the nerves in my leg.

I now cannot stop looking at the pictures that show my very own space invader. It looks huge to me. The radiologist is a very nice man and has given me a sound explanation. Nobody likes to give bad news but he knows that if you hand a brown packet of results to any patient to deliver to their doctor, nine times out of ten they are going to flip the sticky tape and look inside. (I probably wouldn't have done but Roy definitely would have) The radiologist made a very good job of turning a negative into a positive by explaining how operable it would be. He wishes me good luck and repeats over and over, "It's benign Lynda, It's benign".

I did not ask many questions that day due to shock but I am told that research is still going on to find out why people get meningiomas. The only details I personally have read about are that they are usually found in people over the age of 40 and that they are more common in women than men.

MRI Results

Roy and I walked out of that room fast as if we were late to catch a bus. I was aware that my eyes were brimming with tears that I felt I could not yet release. I gripped his hand tightly and tried to stay composed as we walked the short distance to the car. Once in the privacy of our own space I turned towards him and said, "I have a tumour on my brain". After holding tight for as long as we needed he said, "I know and we are now going to make an appointment to get rid of it."

My Brain Tumour

4. Friday 14th July

Back To The Doctors

Let me explain something to you. We know, Roy and I, how to make changes to our lives. We had made big changes to eventually be together. I know that as I sat silently on that car journey to see my own Doctor all my plans and hopes for the future were being challenged. I felt like my hearing and my sight had been temporarily disabled while my mind was churning over all that I had been told.

I decided there and then that this tumour was making an exit and my life was going to continue being as full of sunshine and happiness as it had been over the last two years.

Do not get me wrong. I was scared! Yes I was scared, but I was also determined. My other thoughts included, what happens next, how soon will it take place, where will it happen, how long will it take, are there any after effects and how much will it cost?

How bad could this be? It's benign for goodness sake and it's operable. Let's just deal with it and the sooner the better.

Amazing the mind isn't it? I put it down to self-preservation. If you have something that is fabulously wonderful, why would you let a small hurdle get in the way? Jump it I say and take the challenge!

I can't imagine what was going through Roy's mind on this journey back to see Dr Theophanides. He must have been just as terrified as me but I know he likes to deal with problems head on (so to speak) and that I would draw strength from his positive nature. As we pulled up outside the clinic I knew that we just had to get on with it now and was eager to start the process.

It is strange, but I can honestly admit to being quite an emotional person and if somebody had asked me prior to this how I would react in this situation I would say that I would have trouble keeping myself together and would come out of there without asking any questions.

Well on this particular day I excelled myself. Dr Theophanides looked apologetic – what a job they have! I said I wanted to apologize to him. His diagnosis was right and mine was wrong and that I was very pleased and thankful to have him as my Doctor. I asked all the questions as to what happens next so that I could fit every piece of the jigsaw into place. I had Roy at my side and I knew that he would do everything within his power to help me through. If he had his way he would have taken me straight to hospital and demanded that they remove it there and then so that we could get back to normal the following day.

Things were moving very fast but I'm not sure I needed any more time to think about it. There was only one option in my eyes, so the sooner it was out the better. What would be the point in waiting? It would only allow me time to become scared about surgery details? My options were to fly to the UK and await a place in the NHS schedule anytime over the next 5 years or have private treatment, right here in Paphos, Cyprus. I had no fear of the facilities available here in Cyprus and Dr Theophanides advised me that I would be looked after by the best Neurosurgeon in Cyprus and who is highly respected throughout the world.

This news is very encouraging to me as it means that I would be in hospital not far from home and I was confident in my Doctor, enough to believe him when he tells me they have the right man for the job.

Speaking to him at this time it began to feel quite straightforward and I was eager to discuss what the next steps were. What actually makes me smile a little is that the last time that I was in this man's office I was weeping because he was trying to tell me I should go for an MRI and I was frustrated by what he was suggesting.

Poor Dr Theophanides must have been dreading this meeting and he is such a nice man. He said that he couldn't believe how well we were both taking it and that it made him very depressed to pass on this type of information. I said, "YOU feel depressed?"

Dr Theophanides arranged an appointment for me with the Neurosurgeon for the following day, Saturday 15th July at St George private hospital in Paphos at 11a.m.

The drive home was a little more buoyant and we discussed our joint wish for it to be done as soon as possible. We touched briefly on our fears. Scared because it's a journey into the unknown, it is invasive and it's my head. I am told it is a long operation and I will probably be in hospital for over a week. My added anxiety is that I have never been in hospital before. I am now eager to meet with the Neurosurgeon tomorrow.

My main anxiety of this day was how do I tell my family and friends? Having only lived out in Cyprus for two years all of our very close friends are either in the UK or Australia. My family is spread throughout Europe with my two older brothers living in the U.K. and Spain and my younger sister living in France. This meant that this frightening information was going to have to be relayed by phone and I know that if I had been the recipient of such a phone call, not only would I be shocked but I would want to reach out to support and comfort that person, which is very difficult to do over the phone.

This was not going to be an easy exercise and I needed to think about a plan of approach.

5. Friday 14th July

Informing Family and Friends

What we decided to do was that we should sit down and formulate the questions that we need to ask the Neurosurgeon. We need to be sensible about this, confront our fears and be up front.

What we actually did when we returned home was to make a cup of tea, get on the computer and set about some work. I think we both just needed a little 'time out' to digest what had actually happened to us that morning.

At about 5:00 p.m. we decide to call it a day as neither of us was accomplishing much and we decided to go and sit in the sun outside our local pub, have a drink and write out our questions for tomorrow.

It is quite hard to describe what I was feeling at this time. I was quite hyperactive and felt like I wanted to tell everybody but then not tell anybody. It was a weird time and I felt like all my senses were jumping. I knew I was still in shock to a certain extent because I was also feeling a little weepy.

We had just finished writing out our questions when we were approached by a friend in the pub. Apparently we had been seen coming out of the doctors by a friend of hers the day the doctor had said he wanted me to go for the MRI test. Her friend had said I looked very upset and close to tears and therefore she was concerned that everything was ok.

Roy and I looked at each other and then explained to her that things could be a little better and that I had just received the diagnosis that I had a benign tumour on my brain. Well, that was the first instance of telling someone else and of us seeing the shock expressed by another person. This person doesn't know us that well but we are familiar faces in the pub and often share a joke and a bit of gossip.

Having let the cat out of the bag I then felt the need to share this information. I also believed that if I started informing my precious people it would help me accept that this was reality and not a nightmare.

I decided to phone my best friend Jane in the UK. Jane, Jim and their lovely girls Sarah and Kate had visited us in May that year and we had all had a fabulous time. I knew she was going to be very shocked but I also know she is a brick and her love and support would help me.

I realize now Jane how hard this must have been for you. It did not dawn on me until much later that you were probably terrified for me. A close friend that we had worked with had not survived a tumour three years earlier. I knew the story but did not think for one minute how my news may affect you.

Jane was the first phone call of many that night and they did not get any easier. The cycle of shock continued but what I can say is that at the end of that day I had come to terms with the problem, felt more determined that I would come through it and felt so very fortunate to have such a fabulous group of people that care and love me.

Telling my family was difficult. I knew that I was not going to be able to control myself. These were my siblings and I knew they would make me dissolve into tears which would not be conducive to providing the details and facts in a calm manner.

Roy, once again you took up the task and shouldered their shock. I felt certain that once they had been told and digested all the facts, they would deal with their initial shock and I would be able to speak with them all later. During the course of that evening I did speak with them all. I tried very hard to sound positive and not sound very scared but it's pretty hard to do that when you don't know what is ahead (so to speak). I promised everyone that I would call tomorrow once we had been to see the Neurosurgeon at 11am.

Both Roy and I retired to bed that night feeling mentally and emotionally exhausted and we awoke bright and early the next day ready for the next hurdle.

My Brain Tumour

6. Sat 15th July

Visit To The Neurosurgeon

The date is now July 15th, Saturday and the time is 11am. We have presented ourselves at The St. George's Private Hospital and we wait to see Dr Kyriakides the neurosurgeon.

Full of anticipation, we are led into his office. He asks us to sit down and I hand him the MRI results. I have to say that he is probably one of the calmest people I have ever met. He talks in a gentle manner and studies my face and reactions in great detail.

He asked me exactly what I was feeling and what had led me to visit my doctor in the first place. I explained the symptoms and he said that I have a very good doctor. He wished that more doctors would react like Dr Theophanides and send people for MRI testing at this stage.

Dr Kyriakides then put the images under the wall light in his office and explained in full detail exactly what the problem was and how the tumour was causing a pressure on the brain affecting the area responsible for the nerves in my left leg. He wasn't able to advise why it was growing or what the cause was and said that as meningiomas are slow growing, it could have been making itself known for the last 10 years.

He explains at great length that it is sitting on the top of my brain in the membrane lining. It is not inside the brain itself and therefore it is extremely accessible. He explains that he feels it is a simple and straightforward operation.
At this stage he looked at me and said, "Are you scared?" I said, "Yes, very scared" and he replied, "Don't be scared. There is nothing to be scared about. It's a simple operation and I do many of these each year." He then asked us if we had any questions and was somewhat surprised that we only had thirteen. He patiently went through each one with us, didn't make us feel uncomfortable at any time and in fact, made me feel a lot less anxious about the whole procedure.

I explained to Dr Kyriakides that I was also apprehensive due to the fact that I have never been in hospital before for anything and that probably the worst thing that has ever happened to me was tonsillitis and I haven't even had those removed. He finds this quite amazing and amusing and tells me there is no reason to be worried and that I will be taken good care of.

I studied this man who was to open up my head and make everything good again. He appeared calm and self-assured. I felt that in the course of time this consultation took, all the questions and anxieties had been answered. I knew where I was going, what was going to happen and how long it would all take. It calmed me and gave me goals. Ultimately this doctor exuded confidence and I felt I was in very good hands.

My next hurdle is pre-med checks on Monday 17th July, when I will have an ECG, blood tests and my blood pressure taken of course. I will also be required to have a chest and cranial x-ray.

My Questions & His Answers

Q. How soon will I be able to have the operation?
A. As soon as all pre-operation checks have been carried out to everyone's satisfaction we will then arrange a date to suit us both.

Q. In which hospital will the operation take place?
A. St. George Private Hospital, close to home.

Q. How long will the operation take?
A. As long as it needs to. Usually about 4 hours.

Q. Will there be any pain?
A. No pain.

Q. How long will I have to stay in hospital?
A. Looks at Roy and says, "How long would you like her in there?" Seriously, it's usually between 7-10 days depending on recovery.

Q. Are there any after effects?
A. Highly unlikely. Everything will return to normal and your leg will stop kicking.

Q. Will this operation get rid of it all?
A. Due to the position it is hopeful that I will be able to remove it all intact, however I will not be able to ascertain that until I operate.

Q. Is there a possibility of it growing again?

A. There is a slight chance if all cells are not removed but that is not what I anticipate happening.

Q. What are the causes of meningioma?
A. No one yet knows. Research continues.

Q. Are there any complications with this operation?
A. No more than with any other operation.

Q. What about my hair. Does it need cutting or shaving prior to the operation?
A. Neither is necessary but it is up to you. I will either just simply shave the area where the incision is to be made or a slightly larger area if required. Or if you like I can shave the whole lot.

Q. I have high blood pressure. Will this affect anything?
A. This will be looked at during the pre-operation checks and if necessary will be regulated before and after the operation.

Q. What do the pre-operation checks consist of and when will these take place.
A. You will have a blood test, an ECG, a chest and head x-ray and your blood pressure will be checked. I would like you to see your Doctor on Monday who will make the necessary arrangements for you.

7. Sunday 16th July

A Day To Ourselves

When we left the Neurosurgeons office yesterday I felt relieved. Quite a strange thing to say really, but I say relieved because my questions had been answered and my fears allayed to a certain extent. I now had direction. I knew what my problem was and exactly how it was going to be solved, so my relief was in knowing that there was no longer any guessing to be done, no mind games, no what ifs. It was all there in black and white and now it was just a case of when.

I left the hospital feeling very positive and decided that just in case this was all going to happen very quickly, I would treat myself to a little shopping therapy and go any buy new PJ's and slippers. WOW!

Roy joined me on my shopping expedition and helped with my choice of attire. We also bought a couple of nice steaks and a good bottle of wine and spent the evening at home discussing the next stage.

I had experienced the calm of the Neurosurgeon and Roy and I were not being dramatic which definitely helps. So to those of you out there in support roles, especially large family groups, I would recommend composure because, believe me, I had the googlies screaming to get out just under my skin and I'm not saying it isn't a good thing to express yourself and admit to being scared, which I did, but I didn't want everyone around me flipping out and reacting to me as if I had been given a death sentence. I needed to go to bed and have positive thoughts.

On Sunday we had a leisurely lunch and as it was such a fabulous day, a stroll along the harbour in Paphos. We then returned home and once again phoned family and friends to give them an update on yesterday's meeting with the Neurosurgeon.

Friends and family had digested the information of the day before and it was far more pleasant to have a conversation with everybody in a calm, collected manner. I was able to relate the whole story again and everyone asked the questions that had come to them overnight.

A sense of humour and normality was returning to my world. My sister came out with a cracker when I was telling her about the plans for my hair. I told her that the surgeon had said he could shave the line of incision, shave that side of my head or take the whole lot off if I wanted. She said, "He sounds like a very capable man. Why didn't you ask him if he could give you a perm or highlights while he's at it?"

Roy also came up with a little gem that I decided I would definitely use on the day of the operation. He said, "Ask the surgeon if you will be able to play the piano after the operation. When he says yes of course you will, say, well that's fabulous because I can't play it now."

I also had to shoulder the standard 'lack of brain' jokes from friends and how the surgeon would have plenty of room to work in etc. It was nice to have a laugh again after the last few days of doom and gloom.

On the outside I felt on a slight high but inside I had a personal demon to deal with. My blood pressure problem was definitely going to raise an issue tomorrow and it was my own fault entirely because I should have dealt with this properly a long time ago. My fear now was that it would cause a complication for the operating procedure.

For some reason, unbeknown to anyone, including me, I start telling everyone that the operation will probably take place in about a week to ten days' time. I don't know why or where I plucked this approximation from, seeing as I know nothing about the Cyprus hospital system. Perhaps it just seemed like an appropriate length of time for the tests to be completed and for me to be slotted into the Neurosurgeons diary. How many operations do they do a week, a month, a year? I have no idea, but my tidy mind decides that 1 week to ten days appears reasonable. Figure that one out!

The prospect of waiting this long is quite daunting and although it may give me a little time to plan things, I think, what is there to plan? I was told there was no great rush but it just seems that now that I know I have it, there is very little point in waiting around when I know that the only option I have is to have it removed.

8. Monday 17th July

Pre Operation Testing

The day starts as any other normal day would and it's business as usual in our internet world. Roy and I run a website for villa holidays in Paphos and at this stage we are at a high spot in our season. We have a couple of families arriving this week and others going home, so there is plenty to keep me busy.

At 10:30, we set off to see Dr Theophanides to report back on the visit with the Neurosurgeon. It is decided at this meeting that it will be beneficial to have all the tests done at the same time and in the same place and he places a call to the St. George Private Hospital and an appointment is made for 1pm that day to see Dr Andreas Demetriou. This is excellent, things are moving along well. I have nothing but high praise for my own doctor and the efficiency and speed of the medical services in Paphos. I don't dare express my feelings of how it may have been if I had been faced with the same problem in the U.K.

So, it was home for some lunch and then on to the hospital at 1pm.

I know I am going to have a stumbling block here and I know it is going to be my blood pressure so I had worked myself up about it before we even arrived.

Dr Demetriou explained that I was going to have two x-rays, an ECG and my blood would be tested and typed to ensure that there was sufficient available, if required during the operation. Dr Demetriou was friendly and tried to put us at our ease. He also reiterated that I was going to be in the hands of one of the best Neurosurgeons.

We asked many questions and at one stage received a flippant reply. Roy's anxiety then showed and he became quite frustrated with the doctor who seemed unaware that it was a frightening time for Roy and me. I was told by this particular Doctor that Roy was a worrier and that he worried because he loves me. This was not news to me and I told him so!

I think it served as a little reminder to Dr Demetriou that although he may deal with this sought of situation every day, it is not an everyday occurrence to the rest of us and yes everyone will be anxious and worried and will ask what must be to him the same daily questions.

Then came the crunch time: My blood pressure was taken, I was asked why I wasn't being treated for this, the reading was very high and all my excuses were totally unsatisfactory. I received a good ticking off and deserved all I got but the problem still had to be dealt with. Dr Demetriou advised that until the blood pressure was reduced they would not be able to operate as it would be dangerous. He was therefore going to send me home with an overnight dose of strong tablets in an effort to reduce the reading. In the meantime I was to have the other tests and return to the hospital the next day for another blood pressure reading.

The feelings that are experienced when you let others down is bad but nothing like the feeling that I experienced when I felt I had let myself down so badly that it could affect other people's ability to make me well again. It's not nice. I was angry and very frustrated at myself. So let this serve as a caution to anyone out there who is putting off a visit to the doctors to sort out what you may consider to be a minor complaint. Go now because it could be your downfall at a later stage.

I put on one of the fabulous hospital gowns and had my head and chest x-rayed. No problems there. I had electrodes attached to my chest for the ECG. No problems there. I had blood taken. No problems there and I was assured that there would be sufficient on hand.

So it was now up to me to go home, relax, take the relaxant and the blood pressure medication and return tomorrow for another reading. Relaxing is quite difficult when you are beating up on yourself for being so stupid and I had to give myself a good talking to because some time throughout the course of the afternoon my balance of positives and negatives had shifted heavily in favour of the negatives.

I therefore did exactly what I was told and took the tablets that evening and the following morning and returned to the hospital at 4:30pm the following day.

9. Tuesday 18th July

Blood Pressure Reading

Tuesday was a very long day!
At 4:30 p.m. I returned to St. George Hospital and Dr Demetriou. Yesterday afternoon my blood pressure reading was 170/90. I know this was higher than usual due to the prevailing circumstances but hey, we won't go into that now and start making further excuses. It was high and that was that. Today I am still jumpy and worried because I'm worked up with the expectation. I do in fact have my own blood pressure monitor at home and, of course, I had taken it before I left home – 130/85 which is good for me.

Dr Demetriou takes my blood pressure and is very pleased with the results and with himself. The medication has worked!

"Well", he says. "All the tests from yesterday are good and your blood pressure is now good. I am going to phone Dr Kyriakides, the neurosurgeon and tell him the results of the tests."

The phone call takes place in my presence and I am asked to go home, take the blood pressure tablets for a further night, pack my PJ's and report back for my surgery at:

8 a.m. Tomorrow Morning!

This is really good isn't it? Of course it is. By this time tomorrow I will be able to say, "Well, that's a weight off my mind".

Back at home I started to put all business affairs in order and tried to make things easy for Roy to deal with everything while I'm in hospital. I phoned family and friends to let them know that tomorrow is 'Brain Tumour Eviction day'.

My beautiful little sister informed me that she had found a flight from France and would be arriving in the early hours of Monday morning. This was fabulous news!

My sister Sal has four children, the eldest being eight and the youngest being 15 months old. Sal has not often spent time away from the children so you can imagine the challenge this was to impose, both on the children and their Dad. Her journey was to consist of a four hour train journey to Paris, a four and a half hour flight to Larnaca, Cyprus and then a two and a half hour drive to Paphos. I was quite knocked out that she was doing this for me until I was advised that she was actually doing it for Roy also and herself. She was looking forward to the adventure on her own as it was highly unlikely that it would happen again for a very long time.

I knew she would be great company and support for Roy and provide an avenue for him to vent his fears and anxieties. Knowing my sister, I also knew that she would need to see me herself to be assured that I was in one piece and I looked forward to her making me laugh.

Sally thank you for being there for me. Thank you for making that huge journey and overcoming the frustrations on the way. Brother-in-law, thank you for keeping the home fires burning and affording my sister the opportunity to make the trip. And to Florence, Alice, William and Marcel, thank you for letting me borrow your Mummy for a few days.

I packed my bag, enjoyed a nice dinner, sat and cuddled with my favourite person while watching a film on TV and then retired to bed.

I slept pretty well I think. I mulled it over for a while before sleep, things like how much pain I may feel afterwards and what I'll feel like tomorrow when it is all over and is this really happening to me.

Not much left to say to Roy at this time apart from, 'I love you. I know you will be there for me and it will all be ok'. I know he's scared too and the next 24 hours for him are going to be sheer torture while he waits around for news that the deed has been done and that I have come through it with no complications.

So, as there was to be no further fluids or food after midnight, the alarm clock was set in readiness for another day.

My Brain Tumour

10. Wed 19th July

Operation Day

The alarm sounds at seven and I am out of bed as bright as a button. It is another beautiful day in paradise and the temperatures are already in the low 20's. I make a cup of tea for Roy and shower and wash my shoulder length hair. The thought of not being able to wash my hair again for a while is quite unnerving. I don't want to end up with dread locks and look like 'Sideshow Bob'.

On the way to the hospital it seems as if I suddenly have lots of unanswered questions regarding the smaller details. All the big ones were answered but I wonder how my head will be bandaged, what time the operation will be, how will I feel when I come round and how do they fix the skull bone back? Anxiety setting in I guess.

I am sure I was not alone in wondering whether I was adequately prepared for this brain surgery but I felt confident that the main players were prepared and that they were going to look after me. Positive thinking keeps the mind in focus.

I think I should be nervous, but I'm not. It's strange, but I just want it to happen and after all, I'm not going to know a lot about it during the operation hopefully. I have all the love in the world on my side and I feel wretched for Roy as I know I would be beside myself with worry if the tables were turned.

We are greeted at the hospital by very friendly nursing staff and we commence the standard form filling process. I am advised that the surgeon will be along at about 8:30 to see me. It looked like I was not going to be waiting long. So at the forecasted time Dr Kyriakides arrives and advises me that everything is ready. I will shortly have my pre-op medication administered and I will be visited by the anaesthetist.

I donned my hospital gown, the pre–med was given and I lay back feeling quite relaxed waiting for the anaesthetist. Roy looked far more nervous than me. We knew things were going to happen quite quickly and the air felt electric. Dr Varnavas Papanastasiou, (that is a mouthful whether you are English or Cypriot) the anaesthetist, arrived all gowned up and ready for action, to explain the procedure to me. He had a very confident air about him and a very warm friendly smile and when Roy asked him how long he thought the operation would take he advised about four hours however he had allowed for five. I was suddenly aware that this gentleman was just as important to me as the Neurosurgeon.

The wheel chair arrived and Roy and I looked at each other. He said, "I love you" and I said, "I love you too and will see you soon". As I was wheeled out of the door down to surgery I again heard Roy say I love you but this time it was in Greek. This made me smile because it must have been his way of enlightening the Cypriot staff around me how important I was to him. This fact was to become more than obvious to the various nursing staff on this ward over the next few days.

I was then wheeled down to surgery where I was made comfortable on the operating table. Dr Papanastasiou, the anaesthetist was moving round the top of the table making ready his monitors and Dr Kyriakides, the neurosurgeon was inspecting his tools. The whole atmosphere in the room was one of calm and both were speaking to me and explaining what they were doing and I wished them all good luck.

I decided now was the time to try Roy's joke. I started just as the needle was taking effect and unfortunately I did not see it through to its conclusion. It went something like this:

Me: Do you think I will be able to play the piano after the operation?

Dr Papanastasiou: Oh certainly, you will have no problem with that.

Me: That's amazing, becau…………………………….
(Please see chapter seven for the end of this joke)

Sadly, to this day, they have no idea that I have never played the piano in my life. I knew I'd never make a comedienne, especially if I am destined to fall asleep in the middle of my own jokes.

And so to sleep while the skilled players take to the field and set the world to right again.

I re-enter the conscious world to hustle and bustle where I am aware of people moving me bodily from one bed to another. I can see Roy in the room and nursing staff are attaching me to various pieces of equipment. A catheter is skillfully put in position and a fluid drip is set in motion.

I was lying at a slightly elevated angle and I hear both the Neurosurgeon and the Anaesthetist calling my name and asking if I could hear them. I answer yes and looked at them both standing at the end of the bed. They smiled and then disappeared together. I then see Roy properly as he approached my side with a smile and a kiss.

Roy – I can only express myself in the words of singer 'Ronan Keating':

It's amazing how you can speak right to my heart
Without saying a word, you can light up the dark
Try as I may I could never explain
What I hear when you don't say a thing

The smile on your face lets me know that you need me
There's a truth in your eyes saying you'll never leave me
The touch of your hand says you'll catch me whenever I fall
You say it best when you say nothing at all

I feel very woozy and for the rest of the afternoon I know I drifted in and out of sleep. Every time I opened my eyes Roy was there and I gradually became more aware of my surroundings as the day went on.

There were beautiful flowers in my room and I was conscious of having to stay in the same position due to tubes and wires. There was an incessant beep from the monitor next to me reading all my vital signs, everything being relayed from this irritating peg on my finger.

The most surprising phenomenon to me is that I felt no discomfort or pain at all. No, really, I am not joking. **Nothing hurt!**

At this point in time, I was aware that I had a bandage wrapped right around my head. I was hot but I didn't have a headache. I had a cannula in both hands, one for the drip and the other for medication. I also had a catheter and I had electrodes attached to my chest and nothing hurt. This was marvelous. Was it because I was drowsy, was it because I was numb? I didn't care. Let me wake up gently and if there is going to be pain, let it wait until tomorrow.

What I do know for certain is that Roy stayed by my side all night, sleeping fitfully on a chair while I slipped in and out of sleep and the nursing staff changed drips and administered medication at regular intervals.

For the first time in Cyprus, I saw the sun rise and I was jubilant. Another hurdle over and now it was time to mend. I also had to be brave sooner or later and allow Roy to go home for a shower and to get some sleep. I was in good hands after all, but there is nothing like having someone there who is focused on you and your needs.

Guess What? Still no discomfort and still no pain!

My Brain Tumour

11. Thursday 20th July

Intensive Care Unit

As the day began in the Intensive Care Unit I became very aware of the movements around me while nurses and staff prepared for another day.

I was vaguely aware that I had been tended to at 30 minute intervals during the night by staff checking my monitor, changing fluids, taking temperature and administering medication as I had slipped in and out of sleep and now I was awake, wide awake and actually not feeling too bad at all.

I looked at Roy and it was painfully obvious to me that he had had little or no sleep and had probably been listening to every change in my monitor. I could hear the distant noise of breakfast trolleys and was hungry. Now was the time to get myself together and make Roy feel comfortable enough to go home, shower and work for a few hours.

Like all females beginning to feel on the up, I asked Roy what I looked like, hoping it wasn't too much worse than him. He said I looked a little pail and drawn, had lots of equipment attached to me, had a bandage on my head that looked quite comical AND a tube coming out of my head.

A what?!
A tube coming out of my head??
Where abouts and what is it doing???

I certainly hadn't felt that, though I had been lying in one position all night. This tube was apparently positioned above my right ear somewhere and was obviously for draining fluid which was to be caught in a receptacle on the floor under my bed. This is when you realize how stationery and woozy you have been.

So, on this my first full day in ICU, we both had a cup of tea and Roy set off for home. I was then given a bed bath, clean sheets and had toast and jam for breakfast. The nurses made sure I was comfortable and had everything I needed. I was advised that Dr Kyriakides would be visiting about 11:30 and Roy said he would be back for that. So, until then it was a case of laying back and resting for the remainder of the morning.

At 11:00 Roy was back looking a little more refreshed and Dr Kyriakides arrived at 11:30. He told me he had looked at my records and received a report from the nursing staff and was pleased so far with my progress. He asked, 'any pain or headache?' to which I replied, 'No thank you – do I have to?' He checked my eyes and my reflexes and movement of all limbs. Everything was good. I explained that I felt a slight numbness in my left leg, like a pins and needles sensation mainly around my knee but which could be felt up and down my leg.

Dr Kyriakides advised that this was unlikely to be an effect of the surgery and could be a back problem that was being intensified due to the trauma. What was interesting was the fact that the original kicking and the sensation that this may start at any time that had pre-empted my initial visit to the Doctor, had stopped completely.

He then advised me that he was going to remove this tube, the one that I was totally unaware of, coming out of my head. He was going to nick a little bit of my scalp just to allow free movement and then I would feel him pull twice to release it, which would be followed by two small stitches. At this stage the nurse started busying herself with her trolley, pulling curtains around my bed and asked Roy to leave while they finished. Roy said, 'No' and Dr Kyriakides said, 'it's ok, he can stay'. I wondered if this was a wise decision on his part and if this was to be my initiation to pain.

The scalpel did its job (No Pain!) and then the doctor wrapped the external piece of tubing around his hand, placing his other hand against my head and pulled. What appeared to be an amazingly long piece of tube emerged from my head and then he braced himself and pulled again. I was tensing during this procedure and knew it was all over when I heard a soft pop as the tube made its exodus from my head.

I looked over at Roy; his face looked pretty pale and grim. He was obviously awaiting my reaction and it was easy to turn the grimace to a smile. 'It didn't hurt', I said, 'and these tiny two stitches even feel like pin pricks'.

I really am not kidding you people out there – It did not hurt I promise!

With this little episode behind us the doctor advised that he would be monitoring my progress daily with the nurses and would be back to visit again on Saturday.

I now have total freedom to move my head in any direction I wish and am even able to turn on my side a little to sleep. So with one more hurdle jumped successfully I encourage Roy to go home to get some work done and something to eat.

The rest of the afternoon passes uneventfully. I watch the staff changing shift, I listen to some music and I doze. I receive more lovely flowers and gifts from a friend. The cannula in my left hand feels a little bruised and is becoming uncomfortable when the medication is administered. The nurse inserts a new cannula into another vein to relieve the pressure. It seems the first one had become clogged, as sometimes happens, and this felt much better. At this stage I was really looking forward to when I would be released from all this.

Roy returned after dinner still looking very tired. He had managed about 2 hours sleep but was anxious to return to see how I was. He was such a power of strength to me during this time. He kept a regular check on my drip and my catheter bag and woe betide the nurses if they were unattended to for too long. He questioned everything that was happening to me and made sure that whatever was being done was ok with me. In a nutshell, he was, and is of course, my Mr Wonderful. I'm not sure any of the nurses on this ward had seen such an attentive partner and I was told many times by the Japanese and Chinese nurses how lucky I am. This was no revelation to me. I already knew how lucky I am.

Roy had brought in copies of all the emails he had received over the last two days from family and friends and we read through these together. So many good wishes and funny anecdotes, all of which made us giggle and raised our spirits. It was fabulous to know so many people were thinking about us. I am very lucky to have the good friends that I have and I thank them all for their support. They were all unbelievable:

Jane's Email to Roy said: "Tell her not to fret. She has all the love in the world being telepathically transmitted within this email. I know it's very easy for me to say and not so easy to believe when you have had the world and his wife delving into your head, but all signs are positive and she is on the road to recovery. We all believe it will be ok, because hey, where would we go on holiday next year?"

Ken said: "Pleased to hear she is improving day by day and the panic is over. I take it the fluids she's drinking are non-alcoholic!"

John said: "Please to hear she is progressing well. Tell her we went out with mutual friends last night and of course she was the focus of attention, so at least she has gained some notoriety out of this. Everyone wishes her all their best and we hope to receive a ["made it out in one piece"] email very soon so we can all get back to normality".

Roy decided he would stay at the hospital again that night and as I began to slide in and out of sleep, the night nurse suggested he try and get some rest on the spare ICU bed in the next cubical where he would still be able to hear me if I called. So, he reluctantly agreed and then fell into what must have been the deepest sleep he had had for the last three days.

Well, you may be thinking and quite rightly so, that this has all been a walk in the park up to now, but something is about to change.

I'm not a dramatic person by nature but have never been really good sleeping in unfamiliar environments and as a child was prone to sleep walking which always makes me a tad nervous when placed in this situation. I do not to this day know if this was playing on my mind, especially as I was restricted in movement by being linked to all the monitors or whether I was feeling particularly vulnerable at this stage, but all my calm left me this night and I had an attack of the night frights.

It would seem that every time I managed to get comfortable and fall off to sleep a nurse would appear and would take my blood pressure, administer medication, take my temperature and check the monitors. This was a continual process, which I know was for the benefit of my wellbeing but not conducive to a good night's rest.

The average temperatures in Cyprus in July are 33°C Max and 22°C Min. The air-conditioning in the ICU is running and I am comfortable wearing what can only be described as a very close fitting sock on my head with my hair stuck out the top.

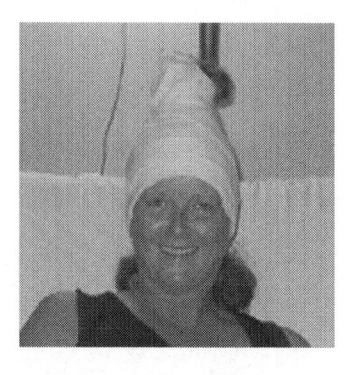

As the night moves on the nursing staff, obviously thinking that I may be feeling a little chilly and to be honest it's not the quietest system I have encountered, so thinking from all angles, they decide to turn off the air-conditioning and open my window while I am dozing. I start to get hotter and hotter. I shed some sheets but am unable to get out of bed to reach the air-con hand set. I try to settle myself but the monitor starts to freak me out because I can see all my reading rising on the screen and the beeping is getting quicker. The problem then escalates out of all control in my mind. The more I get worked up the faster the beeping.

I try deep breathing to calm and control the situation, then I hear a trolley cart down the passageway clanking as if it is being pushed at a fast pace, my imagination takes control and all of a sudden I see myself taking part in the TV show ER and this must be a resuscitation trolley coming for me. The monitor loses it totally and is beeping so fast it goes blank! I call Roy several times but he has fallen into the type of sleep that Sleeping Beauty had when she pricked her finger on the spindle of a spinning wheel and ended up being in that state for 100 years. I press the emergency button that I haven't pressed until now because I'm British and think I can deal with the situation and within a few minutes both Roy and the nurse are at my side trying to calm me down.

My blood pressure is soaring and I feel like I'm having palpitations. I'm wet with sweat, my face is bright red and I'm close to tears. The reason I'm telling you this is because this situation was a real panic for me, I was very scared. I thought I was on my way to having a heart attack. I thought it had all gone horribly wrong and I was going to die – for what seemed like 20 minutes!

BUT, it had nothing to do with my meningioma situation, my operation or my patient care and recovery. This was a trick being played on me by my own mind, my own googlies in the night, my own fears. It can happen! We all fear different things and it doesn't matter how much faith you have in the people around you or how confident you feel that things will work out fine, there will always be a shadow of doubt hiding away in the deep, dark recesses of the mind ready to surface if it catches the opportunity.

The air-conditioning was switched back on, the window was closed, my catheter bag was emptied and I was given time to calm down before being re-attached to that damn monitor. I talked it through with Roy and decided that in the dead of night, when all else was quiet, I was laid awake listening only to that beeping monitor. If the tone changed or something got faster I noticed and it spooked me. He admitted that he had also sat awake the previous night listening to it while I slept and that it had got him going a few times too. We eventually, through total exhaustion fell to sleep – poor Roy on the chair again with his head on my bed.

12. Friday 21st July

Toy Town Ambulance

Well, what a night! It is quite amazing how foolish you can feel after a performance like that. In the light of day I was beginning to wonder what it had all been about and how I could have been so afraid and pitiful. I decided it was time to be rational, put the googlies back in the cupboard and accept that I had in fact had major surgery, was not thinking too straight, it was hot and that damned monitor was getting on my nerves. Enough already and time to move on………….

Roy had several jobs to perform that day to keep our business afloat so left about 10am. He had his mobile phone with him and guess what? No-one seemed to care that I had mine. Maybe it was because I was alone in the ICU. So far I hadn't used it to phone anyone and no one had phoned me – it was only there in case of emergency!

I was monitoring the numbness in my left leg that I had informed the Neurosurgeon about. It was a strange pins and needles sensation that travelled from my knee to my foot and I was happy to go along with the fact that this was probably a back problem as he had explained that it involved a completely different group of nerves. However, I was now experiencing this tingle in my left arm which ran up towards my shoulder.

Now this could have been related to the fact that my arm had been in the same position for a long time or that it was a result of the medication that was being pumped into it, but it was beginning to worry me a little. After last night's episode, I was also beginning to wonder whether I was imagining it. So I tried to relax and read a little to take my mind off it.

The sensation then reached the left hand side of my neck and I really began to feel uneasy. It went away, but when it came back again half an hour later I pressed my call button again and asked the nursing staff to call the doctor. I also at this time sent a text to Roy to come back to the hospital.

Roy returned and I explained what I was experiencing. Having never been through this situation before and not knowing whether I should be panicking or not I decided to err on the side of caution. I didn't see the resident hospital doctor at that time but was advised by the nursing staff that he had decided to take the precaution of having a CAT scan (Computed Axial Tomography) carried out on my head to ascertain if there were any complications. Unfortunately, the CT scanner at the hospital where I was being treated was out of action and they had therefore decided to take me by ambulance to another hospital across town where I had in fact had my initial MRI that diagnosed the tumour. This was ok. I was advised that the same radiologist had been informed and that he would be there waiting for me.

Well this is where the fun starts and I would like to stress at this juncture that what I am about to tell you is a funny story.... Now! I don't want this in any way to detract from the fact that I was looked after well in St. George Private Hospital, but it is something that has to be told as part of my story.

I really have no idea whether hospital politics were involved or whether each private hospital has its own ambulance service that it uses and I do not even want to go into who was supplying the ambulance, but this is what happened and I hope that whatever happened that day has been sorted out and that anyone less well than I was feeling does not have to go through the same performance.

A very nice, polite, older gentleman arrived at my bedside with his stretcher bed and I am aided by the nursing staff to climb aboard. I am now detached from the demon monitor but I still have a drip and a catheter bag to accompany me on my journey together with Roy, of course.

Well, on our way down in the lift this lovely gentleman decides to inform us that he has only recently been employed by the other hospital in town and he wasn't due to start until the end of the month, but they were very short staffed so gave him a call and he wasn't actually sure whether his ambulance was ready yet! I can also advise at this stage that it was likely that he had also not received any gold stars for manoeuvring hospital stretcher trolleys. He did have a very able female assistant with him though who knew the ropes?!

Well the first stumbling block was actually getting the stretcher into the ambulance. He obviously had no idea how to perform this manoeuvre and although I had recently undergone head surgery, my stretcher was pushed back and forth several times before Roy manipulated the tracking and delivered me safely (wait for it!) on board. The young ambulance lady secured the stretcher locking devise, directed Roy to a seat, closed the door and off we set.

We have travelled about half a kilometre down the road and as we swung round a corner the back door on my side swung open. At this stage I am trying desperately to mimic a koala bear and entwine my hands and legs around the hand rail directly above me. I start saying in rather a loud voice that the door is swinging open and although rather startled, the young lady promises me that the stretcher is locked and will not go anywhere.

This is reassuring to note, however, I am not strapped to the stretcher in anyway and want the ambulance stopped. This is when the very nice, elderly gentleman, the driver explains that the mechanic was supposed to have sorted this problem out last week! So the door is secured and we arrive at our destination stressed, hot and anxious about the journey back.

You will be pleased to note out of all of this that the CT scan was clear, the tingling was a bit of a mystery but would be monitored. The radiologist also felt that it could be a back problem and that maybe I would be seeing him at some future date in respect of my spine. For now anyway the head appeared to be great.

While I was undergoing my CT scan, the young lady on the ambulance crew, I was advised later, had refused to travel in that ambulance again, quite rightly pointing out that it was very unsafe and very unprofessional. Great from my point of view but now I have to wait for another vehicle. One and a half hours to be precise! I have now been off the monitor for two and a half hours, nobody appeared to consider that my catheter bag may need changing after this debacle or that my drip bag was also empty.

Never fear – Roy was here! Drawing the attention of the new hospital staff to the fact that they had a patient (whether it was one of theirs or not) awaiting an ambulance for transportation, who needed some attention, they acted quickly. They changed my bag and my drip and even offered me a glass of water. We were then collected by a very professional ambulance crew from the General Hospital who delivered me safely back to where I had come from and the nursing staff were waiting, totally oblivious to what had been happening and enquiring as to whether we would like a cup of tea.

A brandy would have been more apt, even though it was only 3:30 in the afternoon. I felt I had been in a bad dream where Noddy and Big Ears had picked me up in the Toy Town Ambulance and taken me on an exciting adventure that went horribly wrong.

That is enough of all that now. On reflection it is a very funny story to tell. I am quite stunned by what happened and am pleased that I had Roy with me and that I was not feeling very sick. The upshot of this story is that my fears of there being a larger problem were allayed by the CT scan and although the tingling sensation continued I could rationalize that this was probably due to a trapped nerve or a reaction to the antibiotics.

You will no doubt be very pleased to hear that the rest of the day passed uneventfully. Roy returned home and showered.

He returned later, had dinner with me and once again slept on the ICU bed next to me. He had brought fabulous news back with him this time. My sister Sal was coming over from France on Sunday. Now this may not be such a big deal to a lot of you. You may be thinking that France isn't that far from Cyprus, which it's not, but believe me this will have been an army manoeuvre for her and her husband.

Where there is a will there is a way and I knew it was something she had to do, as I would have had to. We lost our parents at a fairly young age and have always been very close. (Apart from when she pinched my white skirt when she was ten that I had planned to wear on the night of a new date)

For the first time since being in hospital, Roy and I both had a full night's sleep. I was still having my medication on an hourly basis, which also involved my blood pressure and temperature being taken, but hey, I'm an old hand at this now and I just ignore them and let them get on with it.

As I slipped happily into sleep, I was pleased to hear my sister was arriving. Roy had been my stalwart and would not relinquish his place as protector and soul mate for anyone. I did not want him to, this is where I wanted him to continue to be but I knew he needed some sleep and he also needed someone to talk to about all of this, to expose his fears and anxieties to and I also felt he was in need of someone else who understood exactly what the fears of this situation were.

The last time they had met properly was when Roy was 15 and Sal was 7. Roy and I having met and fallen in love at the age of 14, at school, were separated by circumstances and spent the majority of our flourishing years with other people. We never lost touch and we met up over the years, if only to remind ourselves that we had always had something special going on. Well my little sister always knew of this bond and when Roy and I finally made it happen three years ago, I am sure she felt like she had known him for years. She was only concerned with my happiness and I was looking forward to her arriving to add her own sense of the ridiculous to all of this.

I knew they would like each other, help each other and forge a new friendship as adults because they had one very important thing in common – ME!

13. Saturday 22nd July

Escape From ICU

Saturday morning I woke up feeling so much better. Surely it must be time to take me off this beeping monitor and let me have some mobility. It would also be very nice to go to the bathroom and enjoy some time alone – how one misses the simple pleasures in life.

Roy was looking a little better for some sleep too and I was happy for him to head off home and return later. He was now beginning to stress a little about my sister's arrival on Sunday late at night. Sally had not made this trip before to our new home and she was to arrive in Cyprus, pick up a hire car and then drive 2 hours to our side of the Island. Her estimated arrival time was about midnight on Sunday. Roy had emailed instructions and would be home awaiting her arrival.

I vaguely remember someone mentioning on Thursday that Lebanon and Israel were on the brink of a war crisis and the nursing staff were reporting a mass exodus from Lebanon to Cyprus as the bombings escalated. I was void of television at this time and until Roy brought in papers for me, was unaware of the extent of the horror.

It was during Saturday morning early that I had my first neighbour in the ICU. He was suffering chest pains and was obviously thought to be on the verge of cardiac problems having suffered the stress and anxiety of fleeing from Lebanon with his family. They had apparently left and boarded a plane with no provisions and only in the clothes they were wearing. The man's wife popped her head around my curtain and asked me if I was aware of any place where she could wash her husband's shirt………..and then apologized when she saw the bandage around my head and the tubes emanating from my body. I was unable to assist her but empathized with her situation and pondered on mine and how we can always find someone in a worse situation.

Later on that morning the Neurosurgeon arrived, Dr Kyriakides. He was very pleased with my progress and now wished to see me out of bed and on my feet. I was eager to comply with his request and managed a few steps down the corridor and back. He suggested I give myself a change of scenery and stay out of bed for a bit and sit on the chair. Not such a big move as I was still attached to everything but a different angle and another great leap in the recovery process.

Dr Kyriakides suggested I take frequent walks, with the nurse's assistance, along the corridor and if I proved to be confident in an upright position with no dizziness then a move from I.C.U. to a private room would be considered for later in the day. Glory be! My own room, my own toilet, my own television, no more peg on my finger, no electrodes on my chest, no catheter bag and no drip. Now let me ask you……how well do you think I did?

I made my escape from the bleeping monitor and found my way jubilantly to the toilet. I donned some underwear and couldn't get out of ICU quick enough and into the corridor. I said to the nurse that I had heard a baby crying in the middle of the night and was advised that there was a premature baby unit very close by. We made our way there and stood outside looking through the windows at the very tiny human beings in incubators fighting for their lives. What a hard start to life. Once again it made me appreciate what I had. Hospital situations certainly open your eyes to other peoples suffering and they can also bring you down if you dwell on them too long. I knew it was time for me to get out of there. I was now beginning to feel like a very well person.

After lunch that day I was given my release from the ICU and I couldn't have been more excited. I felt like an emancipated woman, unshackled from the beeping monitor and liberated from the catheter. Oh, what joy! They even took the cannula out of my arms and I promised to continue drinking lots of fluids.

I picked up my few bits and pieces and with great glee made my way down the corridor to the room that was to become my home for the next few days.

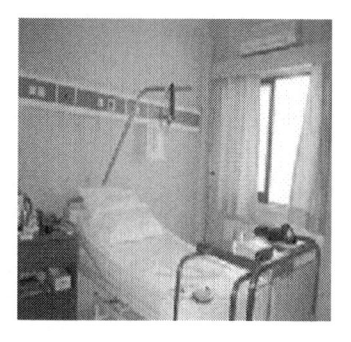

My Brain Tumour

It felt so weird being able to get out of bed when I wanted, watching the world go by out of the window and visiting the bathroom again. My first task was to text Roy to tell him the fabulous news then to take a shower (shear heaven), put PJ's on and butter up the senior nurse to bandage my head again in a more comfortable position for sleeping.

This was all achieved and when Roy visited that afternoon I felt like most of the anxieties of the last few days were ebbing away. The nurses had let some of my, by now, very matted hair out of the hat and I was able to get a brush through it. My head was beginning to itch quite badly which had to be a good sign of healing.

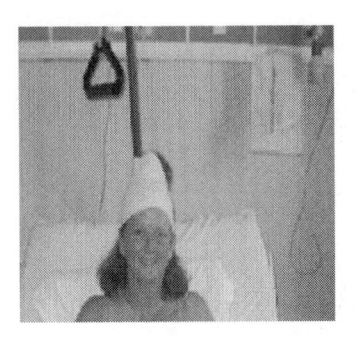

I was surrounded by beautiful flowers; I could now listen to some music on my CD player, watch TV or aimlessly gaze out of the window. It's close to the feeling of arriving at your hotel on holiday and the room facilities far outweighing all your expectations. The only thing that was missing was a mini bar.

Roy stayed and watched a film on TV with me that evening and then for the first time since all this had started he returned home to sleep in our bed. I was incredibly jealous but was actually looking forward to being able to curl up on my side again and strive for a good night's sleep. The nurse advised me that unfortunately the cannula for the intravenous medication should not have been removed and would have to be replaced. The disappointment didn't last long. After all it was only one hand and the regularity had been reduced. I would have my last medication for the night at midnight and then they would leave me to rest until 6am unless I called.

So with that all sorted out, I read a few chapters of my book, closed my door to the ward and drifted off to sleep....zzzzz.

14. Sunday 23rd July

A Quiet Day Of Anticipation

Well I am well rested and awake to the clink of the breakfast trolley at about 6am. The sun is pouring through the window and I feel a surge of excitement at the thought that I am feeling so good, Roy would hopefully have had a good night's rest and that my sister would be starting her epic journey today. If everything goes to plan, this time tomorrow morning Sal should be fast asleep in bed at my place.

The very cheerful auxiliary staff provided me with toast and a selection of jam and cheese spreads and a wonderful cup of tea. Knowing that once they have gone I will not see a warm drink until at least 10am due to showers, bed changing and everything else, I cheekily ask for a pot of tea and coffee and they are more than happy to oblige. Once this had been received, I also asked if it would be a great deal of trouble to have cereals for breakfast tomorrow instead of toast and this was also no problem at all. What a very lucky girl I was – everything was on the up, including me, who only two days ago didn't give a twizzle about what I had for breakfast!

My Brain Tumour

After breakfast I once again sampled the delights of a shower while my bed was being changed. I was pleased that the colour was returning to my cheeks and that the dark circles under my eyes were subsiding. It was still amazing to me that I had no discomfort from the surgery apart from the itching and I was dying to get a look and to know how this would affect my hair. The nurses placed a plastic bag over my cannula hand and basically left me to get on with my shower and enjoy it alone.

The rest of the day was quite hard to adjust to really after the hustle and bustle of ICU days. I got dressed properly and took a walk down the corridor. It was another really hot day and they had opened the door onto the fire escape stairs so I took a sneak out for 10 minutes to feel the sun on my face.

Roy arrived and was beginning to look his normal handsome self again. The dark rings under his eyes were receding and he sounded chirpy. I could put a really awful picture of us both in here just to show you how bad we looked in ICU but I don't know if my vanity will allow it. I'll try it and see......

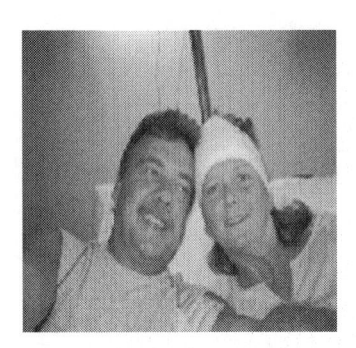

Trust me! We are delirious, hence the stupid smiles. We normally only look half as dazed as this. This brain surgery has obviously affected me far more than anyone expected. It would be unheard of to show myself in public like this – I'm a redhead and I have no mascara on!

A Quiet Day Of Anticipation

Anyway, back to the very exciting stuff....

Tonight's the night my sister arrives and Roy is stressing about her driving in the dark, getting lost and the possibility of his falling asleep prior to the midnight estimated time of arrival, and not hearing her ringing the intercom bell. At this stage I felt it only fair to remind him that my sister was in fact 40 years old, has four children and is very capable of looking after herself. If she gets lost she will just book into the nearest hotel and contact us by phone. So, poor Roy, troubled by the fact that he now has two females to worry about, returns home to await Sally's arrival.

At midnight I receive a text to say, "She hasn't arrived yet!!"

My Brain Tumour

15. Monday 24th July

Sally Arrives

Once again I was woken up early to get my breakfast out of the way. Didn't mind so much today though because I was anxious to hear news from home about Sal's arrival and so excited about seeing her.

6:30 am is a bit early for phoning Roy, so I decide to give my brother a call in the UK, knowing that he would probably just have started work (shift worker). As expected it was 4:30am in his part of the world and he had just arrived at work. He was chirpy and more than happy to have a chat with me.

At 8:30 I phoned Roy, who sounded extremely sleepy. He told me Sally had eventually turned up at 2:00am, having had a night of trauma and having turned the wrong way out of the airport and driven for at least half an hour in the wrong direction. He said they hadn't gone to bed until 5:00am but that he would take her a cup of tea and see if she was ready to wake up. Knowing my sister, as I do, I advised him to tread very carefully otherwise she would rear up like a bear with a sore head and chew his ear off. I suggested he come and see me for breakfast and let her wake up in her own good time.

My Brain Tumour

Well, about an hour later, showered and a coffee shop cappuccino in each hand Roy arrived with a real tale to tell.

In short, Sal's plane had arrived on time but they had been kept standing on the tarmac for an hour waiting to disembark. There were queues due to the many planes arriving in Cyprus as part of the evacuation of Lebanon and the airport was doing their best to process everyone as well as they could. My sister was then faced with an extremely stressed car hire staff member, who by all accounts completed her paperwork and handed her a key and told her that her car was in the car park outside.

None of this fazed Sally until she reached the car park, which is a mini version of any airport car park, in that it has Bays from A through to Z and a multitude of spaces in each. This is midnight in an unfamiliar country and all she had was a key with a registration number on it. The car was eventually located and then as the entire road signs were in Greek, Sally set off in the completely opposite direction. Once she came across a sign post in English and realized she was on her way to the capital, Nicosia, she stopped at a kiosk (late night mini-market) and was assisted by two very nice young gentlemen, who pointed her in the right direction.

You may think that this would be enough for one night but there is more....

Once she arrives at our apartment, she presses the security intercom as directed and guess what? True to all expectations, Roy has fallen asleep and doesn't hear her! This story will be getting very boring to all you readers that do not know my loved ones or the fabulous country that I live in, but just to make the point so that you appreciate my sister's distress, there are no phone boxes around and even if there had have been she had no loose change to phone Roy who had probably fallen into such a deep sleep, he would not have heard the phone either.

Eventually, at about 4:00am Sally gained entry to the apartment, kissed and hugged Roy, put her bags down and requested calmly that a bottle of wine be opened as quickly as possible and that another be put in the fridge to chill!

They managed to turn in at about 5-5:30am, both equally exhausted but both relieved that the journey was over.

After lunch that day, my beautiful little sister arrives and there is much hugging and a few tears but tremendous joy at seeing her smile and listening to her humour while she related the whole story all over again. It was great!

The three of us sat on my bed smiling, laughing and joking as if nothing different had happened in the world. I was very pleased with myself to add my own slice of humour by stating that it was a very sad story and I was so pleased she was here, but truly, on a scale of 1 – 10, how did it compare to having brain surgery?!

I knew that I would probably only get away with that one once and obviously wanted to make it as good as possible. I wanted to sit and listen so intently and emphatically add my Ooh's and Arr's at the right places and then pose the question very seriously. It's very hard (and sad I may add) when you have been waiting a long time with expectation to spring the one liner, especially if you are me. I've never been very good at this sort of thing and I could feel the giggle trying to escape me right from the beginning of the story.

I don't mean to make light of your ordeal Sal. I know you thought my one liner was funny and I will forever be grateful that you made the journey. We needed to see each other and I know you helped both me and Roy just by being you and being there. I love you immensely.

My Brain Tumour

My Sister Sal

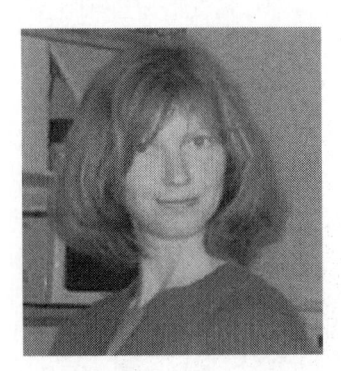

16. Tues 25th to Thurs 27th July

Sally's Stay

These next three days were all about getting better and although I can relate some incidents, none were of a critical nature and most were either funny, emotional or just a joy to experience.

As far as recuperation went, medication was still being administered via the cannula. My blood pressure was still being taken at frequent intervals and everyone was pleased with the results.

I was becoming restless and anxious to be at home on an evening and experience a meal with Roy and Sally. Their paths crossed during the day as they took it in turns to be with me at the hospital. I must have been feeling on the mend because I would have loved to take my sister out and show her Paphos, the harbour and Aphrodite's beach. The closest we got to that was a walk down towards the emergency exit door at the end of the corridor. I wanted to risk the stairs and take a trip to the little shop on the first floor or have a coffee in the canteen but Sal wasn't having any of it.

So over the next few days I caught up on what was happening in her life (she already knew what was happening in mine). We played draughts and generally kept each other company.

Roy managed to take Sal down to the Harbour for lunch so that she at least saw a little more of Paphos than the four walls inside my hospital room. She found the supermarket and cooked a fabulous meal to celebrate the second anniversary of Roy and I being together in Cyprus. We ate this meal all sitting on my bed. The only thing that was missing was a nice bottle of wine... Whine, Whine!

I started to get dressed during the day and taking daily walks around the ward with both Roy & Sally. I was reading more, and one strange thing I found is that just after surgery when I was told not to tax my brain I could do Sudoku puzzles really well. Now that I was nearly on my way home, I couldn't do them and messed them up every time. I'm sure that someone somewhere, if they could be bothered, would have a good explanation for this strange phenomenon but I have a warning for you all out there – Don't attempt them at all or you will end up looking like this:

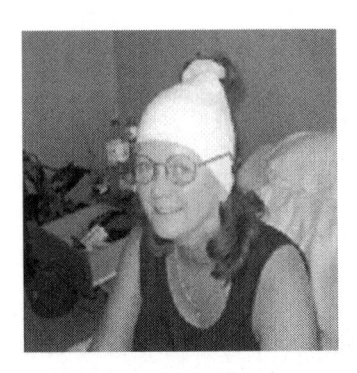

My sister nearly wet her pants when she walked in to the room and found me wearing these glasses. She said, if your skin was blue you could be sworn in as the new member of the Smurfs. Frankly, I have no idea what she is talking about! She then requested that I take them off and be serious as she fell about the room.

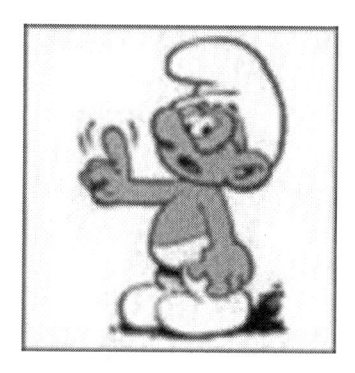

During these few days with my sister, she encouraged me to get dressed, don a little makeup during the day and put some perfume on and generally get back to being myself. Roy and Sal were also there to see the bandage come off and the Alice Band go on to hold the gauze in place. It was such a relief to feel air around my head, to just let a bit of hair free and to comb it.

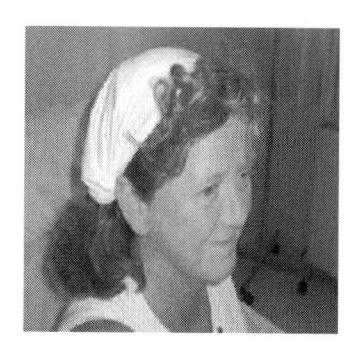

During this week the routine of the recuperation trundled along. I still was woken up at 6:00 a.m. most mornings. Breakfast was good and I was managing lunch most days but it was very special when Sal cooked for me and on her last evening there they brought in take-away. Yummy in my tummy! Sally had asked what I felt like eating and I was desperate for some sort of sauce with my meal so suggested pasta. No sooner suggested than acted upon. They had lasagne and I had spaghetti carbonara and I felt like my taste buds were having a cheerleader moment.

I know that during Sally's stay, the two most important and special people in my life forged a relationship. These two very individual people had met when we were all kids and then again when Roy was 39 and Sal was 30. Although they had spent little time together they should have known each other quite well because they are both a very important and continuous part of my life and knew a lot about each other from me. It may not happen like that for them again, to have to spend time in close company together under stressed circumstances, but from what I have read between the lines from both of you, you did ok! I think you got to know one another properly and enjoyed each other's company and I hope you will feel that bond always.

Sal, your time here was short and I know it was no mean feat making it, but believe that I treasured every moment. I know that it also allowed Roy the opportunity to get some work done and drink more wine in company rather than alone. But all in all the time had come for the reality of life to continue. You had a daughter waiting at home for a birthday party to be arranged, balloons to be blown up, sausages to be put on sticks and fairy cakes to be made and I wanted these stitches out and to make my way home.

We once again said our farewells and promised to meet up again as soon as possible.

To Sally: See my Thank You page.

17. Friday 28th July

Sadness and Elation

I awoke this morning with a mixture of feelings. First off, I was feeling a little down and sorry for myself because I knew it would be another six months at least before I saw my sister again. I was also anxious that she have a better journey home to France than she had had coming here. I knew her little ones were ultimately going to be thrilled to have her home but would probably also be a bit sore at her for going away in the first place.

Now I didn't have the full time attention I really did feel bored and restless. Roy arrived at 8am with fresh coffee and to let me know that Sal was on her way home. I explained how I felt. I hadn't had a doctor near me for days and even the nurses were dropping by less often as the medication and monitoring abated. Surely it must be nearly time to fly this nest.

Then, everything started happening....

A very friendly senior nurse came in to take my blood pressure and to remove the cannula from my hand. Oh joy! No more bags on my hand when having a shower, no more turning over in the middle of the night and knocking it and ultimately, release from one more obstacle that was keeping me here. She explained that whatever medication that was left to administer would be given in tablet form.

"Fabulous", I said "does that mean I can go home today?"
The nurse advised that Dr Kyriakides, the neurosurgeon would be in to see me later in the morning and he would advise me of the next steps. Things were definitely looking up.

At 9:30 sharp, my next visit was the Neurosurgeon, flanked by another nurse and a trolley. Interesting stuff. I was still in my PJ's but my bag was packed (such as it was), magazines and books all neatly stacked and toothbrush and toothpaste stored away in my wash bag.

Ok, I was being a little eager and had forgotten the fact that I still had stitches in my head (I really wasn't kidding when I said there was no pain). Dr Kyriakides told me he was very pleased with my progress. Everything had gone to plan and all that was left was one more day on the antibiotics and to have a look at the wound and take the stitches out. If the wound was good then I would probably be able to go home tomorrow.

Now, never having had stitches in or out before it did cross my mind that this might be the occasion when I may feel some discomfort. I mean, I had seen that Caesarean scar that my sister had. That had been a very neat long line with a bead at each end and they just took the bead off one end and pulled it out in one go. I had no idea how many stitches were involved to start with on the top of my head or the sewing pattern. But, all the nurses, Roy and Sal had said how adept he was with a needle and how neat it was when they had had a peak view while dressings were being changed.

I think it is important to share with you what my head looked like at this time. It may appear shocking to some and I do apologise if you feel this is unnecessary or you are a little squeamish but it does look far worse than it actually was and I do want to emphasize once again that nothing hurt here at all. The scar is horseshoe shaped and although the picture is black and white you will be able to see the long tuft of hair over my ear that is central to the scar line. This surgeon was in fact a gallant marvel who left me with enough hair to provide a covering of this scar for the purposes of vanity and to avoid the heat of the sun.

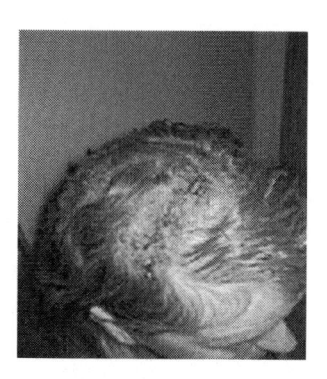

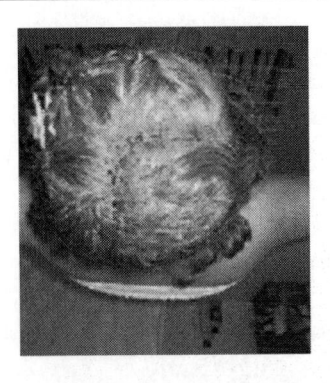

Well they were out in a jiffy and it didn't hurt at all. The scar was all cleaned up, antiseptic was applied and I now knew what was causing all this itching. I now of course had a few questions, the first being when would it be possible to wash my hair and what about using a hair dryer? Would I have to be careful with what products I used and then would there be anything that I was able to do prior to entering this establishment that I wouldn't be able to do now. (Let's not go back to the joke of being able to play the piano)

He advised careful washing of the hair for the first few times while the scarring continued to heal. Then life would continue just as it had before with everyday activities. He suggested that I take things slowly and the only effect to bear in mind was pressure on the skull.

Aah....that would bring me to the next question. We had booked a holiday back in May and were due to fly to Dublin in two weeks' time – would that be a problem so soon after? As it was only a short haul flight he advised all would be ok and the holiday would definitely be good for us both to relax and recuperate.

So at this juncture, I would suggest that while you are on the road to recovery and itching to get out of hospital, ask for a pad and a pen and write a list of questions. It doesn't matter how silly they seem at the time. If you have a surgeon that is as good as mine, they will answer them all and it will stop you becoming anxious once at home. Think about how you think it may change what you do every day. Remember at this stage it is a pressure issue therefore flying should be considered and also I sought guidance regarding my scuba diving.

Anyway, back to my Friday and the next bit of excitement. Dr Demetriou called in next to say how pleased everyone was with my recovery. Dr Demetriou was monitoring my blood pressure and was the unsung hero of my ten day period in hospital. He had successfully reduced my blood pressure sufficiently enough overnight when first meeting me to allow the operation to go ahead immediately. I was also aware that for a small private hospital in the middle of Paphos, he had seen a lot of excitement in the last two weeks with two serious brain tumour treatments causing an added amount of pressure and stress to his weekly load. Dr Demetriou had a look at the surgeon's handiwork, signed me off with the necessary blood pressure prescription and wished me well.

So with all the excitement now out of the way, I settled down to contemplate what had happened over the last 10 days and looked forward to going home. With all my observation results now normal, stitches out and aftercare medication under control I felt as sure as I could be that I was now physically and mentally fit to face the rest of my life. Dr Andreas was interested in the fact that I was writing notes about my experiences. I felt if nothing else it helped me in some way to understand the shock that something like this puts your mind through and how it throws everything in your life into limbo.

I have often heard it said and have even felt it myself after losing a loved one that your priorities change in life. It's good that they do because at some time it is progressive to consider what it would be like tomorrow if things could not be the same. How much of it would truly be important. What should and could we do to make life more enjoyable and should we really wait to do what we desire until we have the time, the money or the guts. It is true that tomorrow may never come and I am not suggesting that we just all drop what we are doing now and go chasing our dreams. But, we should never stop dreaming and every now and then we should take time out to make an effort to attempt them, even if it is in a small way.

So, as you can see, I did contemplate life on my last day in hospital and while I was doing this I also noted an air of relaxation come over Roy. It was like a big sigh of, 'Thank God this is all nearly over, can we please now just go home and start up where we left off'.

I actually felt this was only the beginning of Roy and I expressing our feelings but decided to give him some space to cogitate. He said he was going back home to finish the washing (Bless), pick up a bit of shopping and then he was considering a visit to the pub for a pint in the sunshine. Great idea and he deserved it too. I encouraged him on his way with a huge hug and kiss and knew I would see him later on with news of his day.

It was with great glee and giggles that I received a text from the barmaid in the pub later that day to say she was very pleased that I was due home and that Roy looked so much better and much more relaxed. So relaxed in fact, that he had turned up at the pub in his slippers! What did I say about what was important in life?

I ask you - Does he look bothered?

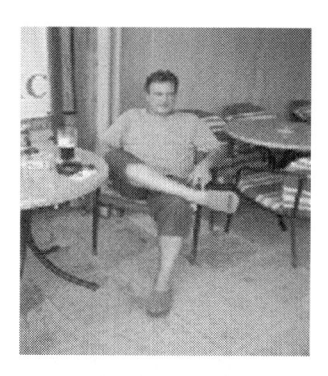

Roy at the Queen Vic – Pint & Slippers. (Isn't it supposed to be Pipe & slippers?)
Thanks for the photo girls.

18. Saturday 29th July

Off Home

Up bright and early, showered and dressed. Makeup on, perfume on and hair brushed as well as it could be. I decided to wait until I got home to enjoy the pure exhilaration of having a shower without being disturbed, running my hands through my own hair and singing at the top of my voice. Oh, was I looking forward to my own environment and my own things around me and the biggest desire was to get into my own big bed, curl up with my lovely man and have a perfect night's sleep, knowing I was back home again.

It did feel strange leaving the hospital and when it came to saying good bye no-one was around. It would appear that these angels were far more important to me than I was to them. By now they had new charges that needed their full attention, just like I did initially. It is fabulous for us that people like them can do the job they do. Tomorrow is another challenge but all with the same routine. It amazed me beyond belief that the young girls that came in to wash me and take my blood pressure in the first few days saw a bandage on my head but actually had no idea what my operation had been until I came out of intensive care. They carried out their duty and care exactly as they were told to do so.

I had just spent, what was to me, a critical and very emotional part of my life in this hospital and it took me all my time to grab Elena, one of the senior nurses for a hug and photo goodbye.

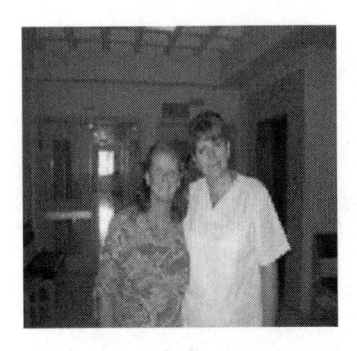

Roy picked me up and off we went home. Nothing to sign, no waving farewells, I was in truth another statistic. All the same, I am forever grateful to the staff of St George's Hospital in Paphos. I was in a foreign country and you looked after me admirably. I have sung your praises on many occasions since and nobody needs fear the expertise and professionalism of the staff in this hospital.

I arrived home to perfect harmony. I know there are females who would have worried about the state of their homes, washing, cleaning, shopping etc. or they would have had a friend call by and help out. I actually knew I didn't need any of this. My little sister had calmed the way when it was needed and remember I had already contemplated what is important in life, yesterday. But seriously, everything was fabulous because Roy is a more than capable human being. The fridge was full, the washing was done and the place was gleaming. Sooooo good to be home.

I unpacked my little case, took a look around and wondered to myself what that last 10 days had all been about.

But first course of action – SHOWER and a SONG!

DEAR PRUDENCE by THE BEATLES

Dear (Lynda), won't you come out to play
Dear (Lynda), greet the brand new day
The sun is up, the sky is blue
It's beautiful and so are you
Dear (Lynda) won't you come out and play

Dear (Lynda) open up your eyes
Dear (Lynda) see the sunny skies
The wind is low the birds will sing
That you are part of everything
Dear (Lynda) won't you open up your eyes?

Look around round, round, round

Dear (Lynda) let me see you smile
Dear (Lynda) like a little child
The clouds will be a daisy chain
So let me see you smile again
Dear (Lynda) won't you let me see you smile?

19. After Effects

I would ask that you try to imagine my relief as life returned to normal for us, but I know it can't be done unless you have experienced it and actually life will never feel exactly the same again because you are jolted into true appreciation of the people around you, the place that you live and the pleasures of everyday things.

I sit here at my computer, twelve months down the track, alive, really well and just about to get married. I have had a follow up visit to the Neurosurgeon. He didn't ask to see me. I just called in to see him on a Saturday morning, 12 months to the day, to take him a bottle of bubbly and to say thanks once again. It took him a few minutes to recognise me! He also said that it was the first time anyone had come back to see him after a successful operation and he was surprised I remembered him!!?? What is that all about?

Remember him! I will never forget him! And let's face it he has seen a bit of me that no-one else on this earth has. I need to keep his number because he is the only one who can truly vouch for the fact that I do have a brain.

My Brain Tumour

On a more serious note, I am now fully fit and healthy. My hair grew back surprisingly quickly. The scalp continued to itch ferociously for many months and still does occasionally. I was told this was the effect of healing and the new growth of hair. Try not to do it too often in public though as it really does look like you have head lice. And be kind to your hair dresser and warn them of the uneven feel and scar on your head. Believe me it's worth it for the extra gentle head massage.

The Neurosurgeon advised me that it was not necessary for me to have any follow up MRI on my head as he had removed all sign of the tumour. So that was it, all finished. I had a brain tumour, a short spell in hospital and then it was gone. No after effect and no continued medication but you know me now and I haven't really changed a great deal from when you met me at the beginning – I don't like to leave things to chance.

It's not that I don't believe my Neurosurgeon but like many of you out there, I have read other people stories on the internet. Everyone has a different tale to tell and I will be paying for a follow up MRI occasionally just to keep them demons at bay because if I ever have to deal with space invaders again I want to be ready to attack them early.

There is one little thing I will clear up now though that may have been a little confusing throughout my story and was in fact a red herring. Do you remember right back at the beginning when I thought the involuntary spasm in my leg was a back problem? Then whilst I was in intensive care I had the tingling in my leg, which at one stage crept up my arm and into my neck. It frightened me so much that they took me in the Toy Town ambulance to have a CT scan. Well, you will be pleased to know that I got to the bottom of that one.

This tingling sensation and overall weakness in my left leg did not cease afterwards and I just became used to it. Six months after the tumour operation I decided to put a stop to the niggling doubts in my mind that surface from time to time and go and have it checked out properly. I had an MRI on my spine. Don't let your imagination ever get the better of you – it is the land where nightmares are manufactured.

There were no tumours to be seen in this area but I did have a disc problem in my lower back. This disc problem was the cause for the nerve tingling, which was obviously highlighted due to my lack of movement in ICU. I have no pain and the numbing effects have diminished to a state where I hardly notice it anymore. You see, I am able to put this into a small place because I now know what it is. It is the fear of the unknown that drives us mad so it's always best to check things out.

Since starting this E-book I have heard many stories of other people's experiences and I even met another survivor two months ago. His story and his journey were very different from mine, but the end result was the same, I am very pleased to report, as he is now fit and well.

Before my brain tumour diagnosis I had not met anyone who had had the same or similar tumours and therefore I was unable to draw on anyone else's experience or assurances. In the few afternoons that I had after being diagnosed and before going into hospital I sought as much information as I could from the internet and devoured everything I read. But, a great deal of the information on the internet is aimed at the medical professional and not the victim. I went into forums looking for a story like mine and although I was very touched by the support that these groups provide, I was also very depressed because it was very infrequent to find a happy positive ending to most of the reports.

I therefore decided to set about offering a balance in this book. I know that everyone's story is different, some brain tumours are more serious than others and there are many outcomes. I want people to understand that there is often a happy, positive result and that many people are given a second chance, like me.

I don't want to mislead anyone and it would be crass of me to say that it is not a serious diagnosis. The surgery is intrusive and the emotional roller coaster ride is probably the biggest nightmare everyone around you will endure but there are not enough happy endings out there in print. It would have really helped my state of mind to see a few more and to know that there can be light at the end of the tunnel. Because of this I have entered the forums and tried to tell my story too so people will not feel totally discouraged.

I really hope that by reading this book, whether you have been diagnosed or whether you are a family member or friend, it will give you a small window in to the procedure and an insight into what to expect and how everyone is going to feel.

I don't believe for one minute that anyone can adequately prepare someone else for a brain tumour operation. As I said in the beginning, the words themselves strike fear into the pit of your stomach and I know it stays there until it is all over. You know that whether you feel really bad or really good, like I did, at the time of your pre-med injection, there is a true possibility of a horrible outcome.

You could go down the route of Ronan Keating's song, 'If Tomorrow Never Comes', I personally didn't go there and my mind must have shut out that possibility because I believed that I could meet any obstacle that was challenging my happiness. No one had a bigger desire to live than me. My life was the happiest it had ever been. My big frustration was that this was out of my control. I'm not a religious person but I left all options open that day. I am grateful for being given another throw of the dice.

The point is, there are a myriad of places on the net with information, some informative if you have a medical degree and some very discouraging. I have dedicated a chapter to resources for you to obtain well balanced facts together with other stories from meningioma survivors.

I wish you all out there lots of Good Luck on your journey!

I would strongly recommend that if you are in a country and area that has a brain tumour support group, to join them. Sharing experiences with others not only helps you to understand your own fears and problems but will help you to learn and help others in their journey.

Quote by Ambrose Redmoon - "Overcoming Adversity"

'Courage is not the absence of fear, but rather the judgment that something else is more important than fear'.

OUR WEDDING DAY

29th February 2008

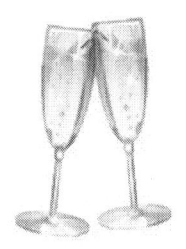

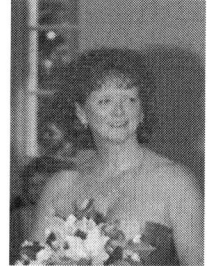

It's Not A Hat – I Promise!

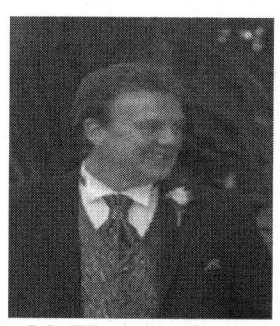

My Hero Husband

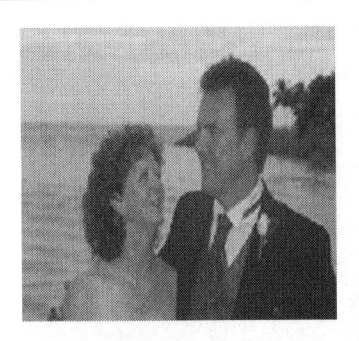

QUOTE: From Love in the Time of Cholera
by Gabriel Garcia Marquez

'It was a time when they both loved each other best, without hurry or excess, when both were most conscious of and grateful for their incredible victories over adversity. Life would still present them with other moral trials, of course, but that no longer mattered: 'They were on the other shore'.

My name is now Lynda Carter (nee Burke).

For those of you too young to remember, Lynda Carter played 'Wonder Woman' in the fantasy-adventure TV series which aired from 1975 to 1979 and I am happy to try and live up to the name.

Lynda is donating a percentage of every sale of her book to meningioma research.

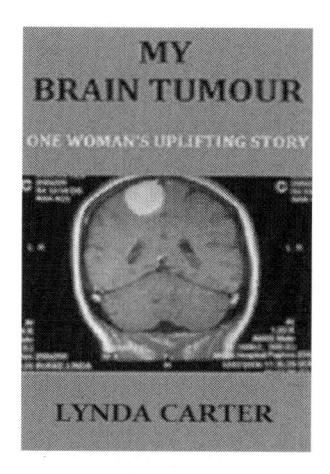

MY BRAIN TUMOUR
ONE WOMAN'S UPLIFTING STORY

LYNDA CARTER

My Sister Sally's Version Of Events

I felt like Zinadine Zidane standing there in the concrete car park. Exactly 2 weeks earlier, Frenchman Zidane had, with his team, battled to reach the Football World Cup Final only to be beaten by the Italians. In these wee small hours my journey's end found me in something of a predicament. I could not complete my long journey unless I got an answer from this apartment block door.

Zidane was not gracious in defeat, and neither was I. The quiet of the warm Paphos night was assaulted by my ringing, knocking, banging, shouting and bawling. Nothing. His car was one of the three cars parked in the small car park. The engine was cold. There was no sign of a phone box, and even if I had found one on my drive round the dark unfamiliar streets, I had no Cypriot coins. In addition to the exhaustion he must be feeling, he is also a known offender of the mutton Geoff (deaf) variety.

How to wake Roy?

My Brain Tumour

With my husband and children, I had spent the weekend of the world cup final with Scottish friends who have a holiday house about half an hour's drive from where we live in south west France. On the road homewards, while our 4 exhausted children and dog slept, my husband John and I chatted affectionately about the wonderful time we had all had. Temperatures were in the 40s; we had camped in their garden and watched the football match on a large outdoor screen in the middle of the village. All evening packs of liberated children, ours included, ran with abandon. The French do these occasions well. We had all stayed up too late, drunk too much wine and had had a rip-roaring time. It didn't seem life could get any better.

At home, our then six year old, Alice, had taken on the role of telephone receptionist. In part this would be a normal part of her development but she has been actively encouraged because her French is so much better than mine. So she took the call.

"Who was it, Ali?" I said from the kitchen.
"It was for Daddy, not you."
"OK, but who was it?" becoming slightly exasperated.
"Roy, but he only wanted to speak to Daddy!"

Boom, boom, boom, boom. My heart forgot how to beat with the right rhythm.

John, my husband, was in town, so I passed an hour of what I can only describe as torment.

A car crash, a stroke, a mugger, he had done it, he loved her so much, you have no idea what was going on in my head. But anyway, she was definitely dead. So how would they break the news and how would I receive it. On feeling that my life had become unreal, it's amazing how my brain adapted to madness. I was coolly planning the funeral when John arrived home. While he was on the phone with Roy, I sat in the shade of the horse chestnut trying to remember how to breathe. I think I actually received the news about the tumor with incredible calm and attention to detail. Not that surprising really, given the scenario I had previously invented.

The children could have had fish fingers for tea, and frankly would have preferred them to the elaborate chicken casserole with which they were presented. However, fish fingers would not have provided me with the excuse to be a martyr. A weary damp wipe of forehead with back of hand, while chopping onions and garlic, and I could believe 'I must provide goodness for my children before allowing any attention to my own feelings'. In fact, this normalness of life gave me time to digest the information before I made that very scary call to Lyn. The thing about sisters, who are close, is that they suffer a destructive instinct to second guess each other. The reason this is destructive is that though their guess may be well founded in their shared history, as the song goes 'it ain't necessarily so.' The responsibility, to respond in the way one feels the sister needs, is intense.

With eight years between us, my sister has been many people to me. As a child I remember feeling competition for Mum's affection. My friends, and I, watched open mouthed and adoringly at her sophistication, her make-up, high heels and social life. My beautiful, popular, clever big sister. It was my sister who told me about periods, my sister who I wanted to rescue me from my boarding school and my sister who explained to me that my first love, a dashing RAF pilot, was, in fact, not visiting his sister every weekend.

So I have the information. I pick up the phone. I dial the number. We talk. I ask questions, she answers. We are very grown-up. And then I revert to type. I am 13 once more.

I don't remember how the rest went, too much wine has a way of protecting you from memories, a decent Chablis as I recall. We called it injustice, we based ourselves in our history and we cried. I promised that she would not be alone through it.
"I'm not alone", she said.

Although she felt the operation was imminent, she did not have a firm idea of when it would take place. Should I follow instinct and leave immediately then have to leave before the operation? Should I wait to discover it was all over, I'd be more use afterwards – we didn't talk openly about what the outcome could be. It was implied. John and I are occupational therapists and this gives us enough information to be depressed, not quite enough to be re-assured.

That evening, John sat through my irrational laughter, rose-tinted past and uncontrollable sobbing. It was agreed that I should go to Cyprus as soon as possible. We were really struggling financially so I trawled the net, spoke with friends who work for airlines and decided to travel via London, as any flight direct from France was extortionate, especially at such short notice. I had booked the first leg, La Rochelle to Gatwick, when Lyn called to say she had been for another consultation and would be seeing her consultant again the following weekend to get a definite date for her operation. She recently told me that she has no idea why she told me this, and that she really knew what was going to happen. It might have saved me a euro or two if she hadn't.

I cancelled the flight to Gatwick and started to plan to go in the following week. Finger poised on the 'buy' button, I received another phone call telling me the operation would be the next day! Having cancelled the Gatwick flight, I now couldn't get another for that day. I had to swallow my own frustration and feelings of panic and powerlessness, because this was not about me. Lyn and I talked on the telephone that night before the operation. I couldn't say what we talked about. I hope I was supportive. It was a horribly necessary contact. It is just not possible to give a fully effective cuddle over the telephone.

I borrowed money from my childhood best friend, Janie. Incidentally the same friend who helped me test my big sister's new platform shoes for water-tightness down by the river. My journey of literally planes, trains and automobiles began within 48 hours.

On the train to Poitier, I sat still in shock. I was leaving my very young family for the first time, to go on this long complicated journey on my own. I was so self-absorbed, I think with fear, during the journey that at times I acted uncharacteristically. I changed trains in Poitier to find my seat taken by a middle-aged couple clearly enjoying each other's company. I thought of Lyn & Roy, so not wanting to disturb them, I sat in a spare seat close by. At the next stop, the rightful owners of my current seat got on, and the train was now full. Ordinarily, I would have responded to the situation with generosity towards the couple in my booked seat but today I didn't want to stand all the way to Paris so I told them to move. I felt slightly bad but hell, I'd never see them again.

My eldest daughter, Florence, is a very popular member of her class at school. She gets invited to every birthday party. She has Down's syndrome which does not in any way dampen her social life. This fact is only important to this story because her birthday happened to be involved. Before the end of the summer term, she had invited to her birthday party, her entire class. Although daunting, this would not usually be a problem; we have a large garden and the French summer is guaranteed.

The practice here at birthday parties, whatever the age of the child is to drop them at the gate and scarper. So John was looking at being left with our 4 small children for the first time, for at least a week, and on top of that hosting a 7 year olds birthday party for up to 25 French children, on his own! The party could not be cancelled as the invites had been given out at school, the French do not RSVP (ironically) so we had no way of contacting anyone. It had to go ahead.

So best foot forward, I traversed Paris and got on the direct plane to Larnaca. Interestingly, I saw the French couple that I had moved from seats on the train in the check-out queue. This flight coincided with the terrible crisis in the Lebanon, when all people who could travel, were also heading for Cyprus. On the plane, I was sat next to a young Cypriot chemist who was amiable enough to translate for me, the pilot's discussion, as we sat on the runway with several hours to wait to clear customs. Apparently, there were seven planes ahead of us waiting to unload, but as it turned out, our pilot, a Cypriot, was a cousin of the controller's sister in law, so our plane got bumped to the front after only an hours delay on the tarmac. We had been told to expect a lot longer. She (the chemist) said "Oh that is so Cyprus."

Now although this plane queue jumping, worked in my favour, I felt very afraid for my sister. If that's so Cypriot where does that mean she comes? End of the list?

It was so busy at the airport; the car hire place threw keys at me and gestured in a general direction north. The French couple were there too! They seemed to know where to go, so I surreptitiously followed them. It was 11pm and I then spent an hour trying these keys in each small car, enclosed in a large unlit field, until I found one that fit. Two years later, no-one has reported the theft, so it must have been my hire car.

I set off from Larnaca focusing on seeing my sister. Lucky for me, Roy had emailed me idiot proof directions straight to their door. Unfortunately, he had forgotten to mention that my first target 'head towards Limassol' is usually on signposts, in Greek as 'Lemesos'. After my detour via Aiya Napa (at the opposite end of the island) I eventually had to stop off at a small, incredibly open, 'shoppette' where various young men were drinking chocolate milkshake, in their pyjamas, to ask for help. Armed with their information, I found my way around Limassol and Paphos no problem. At least, no problem except for the fact my hire car had no dipped beam, it was sidelights or full. Actually, I didn't care about the people driving towards me, I was on a mission.

So here I was, trying to wake Roy.

I did wake Roy eventually, poor love, the first time he'd slept in days! He made me feel at home and filled me in on events so far. That night, I felt my heart tear for him. He was being everything for Lyn. A rabbit caught in headlights would be easy to describe. Roy was a gazelle in stasis. He had been everything and done everything right, and I didn't really know him. Our evenings after the daily hospital visits would soon change that. It was an amazing opportunity to get to know the man my sister loves, without her getting in the way. He had not slept in over a week.

It was almost morning when I arrived, so it would be the next day before my sister and I would see each other. Roy took me in to the hospital, drove like a crazy man – but apparently that's normal for him. I saw my sister in bed with the funniest hat on I have ever seen.

Sally's Version Of Events

Me and Lyn have a history of amusing events, so thank God, her bandage was funny. We had a very tearful, serious first hour, and then I had to say, 'now take that bloody silly hat off'. The 'hat' provided much amusement, daily. I'm not sure it was necessary medically; I truly believe it was there to provide a smile.

In the week that I was in Cyprus, I trod a line that never felt uncomfortable. I wanted to be with my sister, but I didn't want to impose on her time with Roy.

Actually it was nice to feel a bit like a distraction, giving light to her and allowing some sleep for him. Looking back, I have no regrets about my actions. It was important to be with my sister, regardless of how I tussled with myself about leaving my children. I knew they would be fine but it was still hard to do.

Those days in the hospital were surreal. Normally, no two people would spend that quality of time together. I myself am shocked to say, given the circumstances, we laughed so much. I think it may have been the second or third day; Lyn was clearly exhausted, I suspect I had added to that.

I was there with my sister enjoying seeing her get better. Fate had kept me away during the operation, but I was so glad to be there, seeing her get stronger everyday. I was living in her home, while she was in hospital, and I ached for her to be there too. I was incredibly sad to leave before she was discharged from hospital, but I was no longer worried. It was the best time to have spent together, when she was scared or worried or happy to look forward again, I was there to share those hours with her.

I left Cyprus with an uplifted heart, Lyn still in hospital, but discharge was imminent. Whatever happened now could not be anywhere near what we all had first thought. That was until we hit turbulence coming down in to Paris and the plane simply dropped 30 foot. I yelped liked a kicked puppy, and then really, really cried. The calm hefty Cypriot man sitting next to me clasped my hand and said 's'orright, s'gonna be orright.'

MY THANK YOU PAGE

It is really hard to make sure you don't forget someone when you say 'Thank You', which sounds so inadequate anyway. It is certainly a time when you truly find out who your close friends are. It's like shaking a jar of oil and water. You know you have lots of good friends in life and we all have our own routines, troubles and agendas. The water bubbles struggle to the surface showing they are different. You all know who you are and I promise you all to be the bubble of water that fights my way to the surface. I will be there for you if ever you need me.

I am grateful for being given more time to fulfil my dreams. I have to add that I can't listen to the Ronan Keating song anymore without a lump in my throat and a tightening of my chest and I promise to let my loved ones know every time I speak to them how much I love them.

The friends and family below deserve special mention because of funny or touching things that happened along the way. Roy & I thank you. We feel privileged to have your friendship.

*"Friends are like bras –
close to the heart and there for support"*

Jane Garnham – You are my best friend through thick and thin. You make me giggle, you make me feel courageous, and you make me feel strong even when you know I'm not. You make me feel everything a best friend should make her friend feel. Thank you for being my test pilot when I had to spread the word. I promised to share the happiest times in my life with you as well as the worst so thank you for travelling all the way to Australia to be at my wedding.

Ken & Jane – You are my friends of old and we share a lovely bond. You took my man under your wing even though you had never met him. You shared your humour with him throughout and I am indebted. He now realizes why the friendship has lasted the test of time and separation.

Kev – I'm so pleased you started work at 4am. I enjoyed our talk so much and I'm so pleased you were the first to hear how fabulous I felt.

Dan – I'm sorry I couldn't get hold of you initially in Spain but it was good to know that the guy who did keep answering your old number had the grace and patience to listen to my joy about going home – Even though it was 6am.

John & Maureen – Maureen, thank you for finding the only soft teddy with a bandage over his head and John, your support to Roy, I know was priceless. I'm sorry I woke you with my phone call at 4am I forgot the time difference. I was on a roll!

Sarah & Kate Garnham – Your daily texts kept me going sweethearts. I love you.

I am indebted to the following people:
Dr Chris Theophanides. If it wasn't for you, I am aware this whole experience could have panned out very differently. Thank You.

Dr Christos Kyriakides, you are one of the most unassuming men I have come across. You are calm, you are approachable, and you have hands that save lives. You are my super hero.

Dr Varnavas Papanastasiou, you are professional, warm, friendly and caring. You are also my hero.

Dr Andreas Demetriou and The staff and nurses at St. Georges Private Hospital in Paphos – you looked after me admirably.

TO SALLYANNE (*My Beautiful Sister*)
QUOTE: *I feel a very unusual sensation - if it is not indigestion, I think it must be gratitude. ~ Benjamin Disraeli*

My sister often held my hand
When she was very small
I took the time to help her out
And I did not mind at all.
My sister came and held my hand
When I felt small and scared
She took the time to help me out
And she did not mind at all.
My sister is a blessing
And I love her everyday
Thank you for being there for me
I really appreciated your stay.

I love you.

TO ROY – Words cannot express my love for you!
'Piglet sidled up to Pooh from behind, "Pooh", she whispered
"Yes piglet?"
"Nothing", said Piglet, taking Pooh's paw, "I just wanted to be sure of you".'

This is my wish for you: Comfort on difficult days, smiles when sadness intrudes, rainbows to follow the clouds, laughter to kiss your lips, sunsets to warm your heart, hugs when spirits sag, beauty for your eyes to see, friendships to brighten your being, faith so that you can believe, confidence for when you doubt, courage to know yourself, patience to accept the truth and love to complete your life.

If ever there is a tomorrow when we are not together, there is something you must always remember .... You are braver than you believe, stronger than you seem and smarter than you think. But, most of all, even if we're apart, I'll always be with you.

Life is a journey, and love is what makes that journey worthwhile.
The journey is the reward.
I wonder if you'll ever know how much you mean to me,
For you have made me realise how happy life can be.

I have seen you a million times
And every time I see you
I fall in love with you all over again
My heart starts to race
My frown turns into a smile
And all my worries are now in my past
When you smile at me my heart melts

Your smile is like a new day
Your sense of humour is like no other
The ability you have to make me smile
Is all you need to love me
Just looking in your eyes
Makes me melt inside

I love you.

Some Facts And Resources

A meningioma is a tumour of the meninges, which are the protective membranes around the brain and spinal cord. Malignant meningiomas are extremely rare. Most meningioma's are found to be benign. Meningioma's make up nearly 1 in 5 of all primary brain tumours and are more common in women than men.

Causes of a meningioma
As with most brain tumours, the cause of a meningioma is unknown. Research is being carried out into possible causes.

Your Meningioma Diagnosis
http://www.boston-neurosurg.org/publications/YMD.doc

The following websites are very much up my alley. They offer hope, sensible advice and some fabulous success stories. Liz from Meningioma Mommas makes a very important point on her front page, 'Even though we all have compassionate spouses, family members, friends and caregivers in our lives, we often find it's much easier to share our concerns, fears and doubts with those who've walked in our shoes'.
http://www.meningiomamommas.org/
http://www.getyourheadinthegame.org/support/survivor_stories.php

Worldwide Resources
http://www.cancerbackup.org.uk
http://www.braintumouruk.org.uk/

http://www.braintumouraction.org.uk
http://www.mywavelength.com/index.php
http://bta.org.au
http://www.carepages.com/
http://www.tbts.org/
http://www.cancer.gov

QUESTIONS FOR THE NEUROSURGEON

Preparing for Treatment
These are some questions a person may want to ask the doctor before treatment begins:
- What type of brain tumor do I have?
- Is it benign or malignant?
- What is the grade of the tumor?
- What are my treatment choices? Which do you recommend for me? Why?
- What are the benefits of each kind of treatment?
- What are the risks and possible side effects of each treatment?
- What is the treatment likely to cost?
- How will treatment affect my normal activities?

Before Having Surgery
These are some questions a person may want to ask the doctor before having surgery:
- How will I feel after the operation?
- What will you do for me if I have pain?
- How long will I be in the hospital?
- Will I have any long-term effects? Will my hair grow back?
- When can I get back to my normal activities?
- What is my chance of a full recovery?

Radiation Therapy
These are some questions a person may want to ask the doctor before having radiation therapy:
- Why do I need this treatment?
- When will the treatments begin? When will they end?
- How will I feel during therapy? Are there side effects?
- What can I do to take care of myself during therapy?
- How will we know if the radiation is working?

- Will I be able to continue my normal activities during treatment?

Chemotherapy

Patients may want to ask these questions about chemotherapy:
- Why do I need this treatment?
- What will it do?
- Will I have side effects? What can I do about them?
- When will treatment start? When will it end?
- How often will I need check-ups?

Note From The Author

If you have enjoyed reading this book and think that brain tumor sufferers or their family and friends may benefit from reading it please kindly take a few minutes and return to Amazon and leave a review. Your time is much appreciated:

http://www.amazon.com/dp/B0044R9DDU

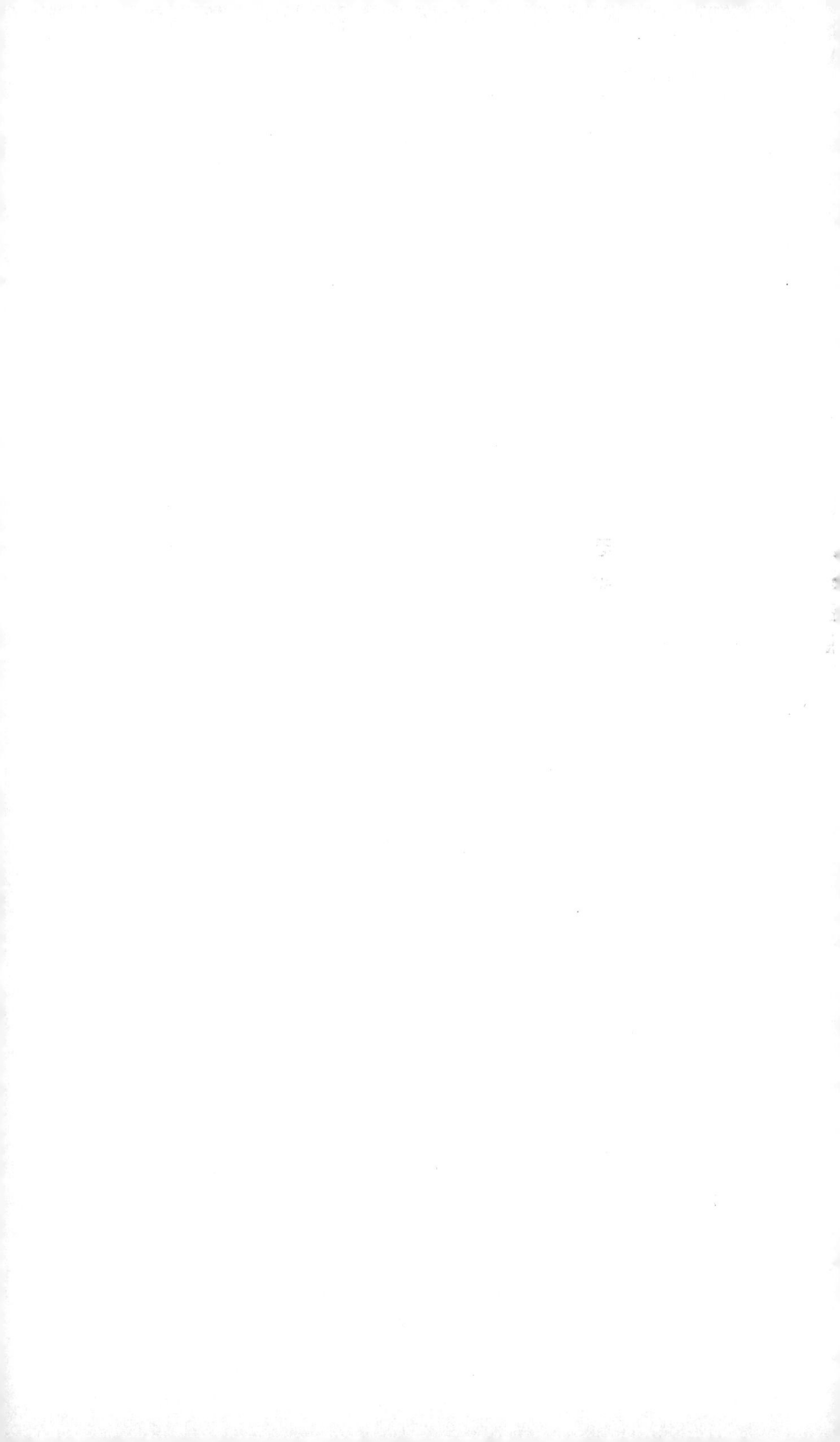

Made in the USA
Las Vegas, NV
01 November 2021